A PRACTICAL GUIDE TO
WORKING WITH
PEOPLE WITH
LEARNING
DISABILITIES

A handbook for care assistants
and support workers

Edited by
Hilary Brown
and
Sue Benson

HPL

First published in 1992 by
Hawker Publications Ltd
13 Park House
140 Battersea Park Road
London SW11 4NB
Second Edition 1994
Second Edition (Revised) 1995

British Library Cataloguing in Publication Data

A catalogue record for this book is available
from the British Library

ISBN 1-874790-12-4
(First Edition 1-874790-00-0)

Designed by
Richard Souper

Typeset by
Hawker Publications

Printed and bound in Great Britain by
Butler and Tanner, Frome, Somerset

*We would like to thank Glenn, Mandy and the staff of 175 Maidstone
Road, Chatham, who appear in photographs on pages 63, 84, 125 and 151,
and Ken Dickson who appears on page 91.*

Other titles in this series:
Handbook for Care Assistants – A Practical Guide to Caring for Elderly People
Fourth Edition 1995. ISBN 0-1-874790-19-1 Price: £14.95
The Handbook for Community Care Assistants and Support Workers
1995. ISBN 1-874790-18-3 Price: £12.95
The Care Assistant's Guide to Working With Elderly Mentally Infirm People
1991. Reprinted 1993. ISBN 0-9514649-6-5 Price: £9.95
The Handbook for Hospital Care Assistants and Support Workers
1993. ISBN 1-874790-10-8 Price: £9.95

Contents

Contributors

Sheila Barrett is Lecturer/Service Development Consultant at the University of Kent, and has spent many years developing services and staff competencies in challenging behaviour.

John Brennan is a Senior Social Worker with the Medway Community Living Service, involved with the closure of long stay hospitals for people with learning difficulties.

David Brooks is Consultant in the Psychiatry of Mental Handicap with Bexley Health Authority. He teaches on the programme for the Diploma in the Applied Psychology of Severe Mental Handicap (Challenging Behaviours) at the University of Kent.

Hilary Brown is Senior Lecturer in Learning Disabilities at the Tizard Centre at the University of Kent at Canterbury. She is currently directing a research programme funded by the Joseph Rowntree Foundation on the sexual abuse of adults with learning disabilities.

Anne Clarke-Kehoe is a speech and language therapist whose particular interests are people with profound multiple disabilities and those whose behaviour is seen as challenging. Previously manager of a speech therapist service for special needs clients, she now works as a freelance trainer and consultant.

Peter Ferns is an Independent Training Consultant with many years experience in care for adults and children with learning disabilities. He provides consultancy and training in the areas of learning disability, mental health and community care management issues. As a Black trainer he has been involved in many initiatives on race equality in social work.

André Fox RNMH is Community Service Manager with the Medway Community Living Service which provides health care and promotes independent life for people with learning disabilities.

Liz Garnham Hooper is Head Occupational Therapist for learning disabilities in Richmond, Twickenham and Roehampton Health District. She has trained in the USA with Marc Gold and Associates.

Pauline Gee RNMH is Settlement Coordinator for Camberwell Health Authority Learning Disabilities Care Group.

Liz Henderson is an Employment Worker for Alpha Employment in Kent, supporting people with learning difficulties in work opportunities.

Mike Higgs RNMH is a Day Centre Manager for Haringey Social Services. He has worked both with people with learning disability and those with mental health problems.

Heather Hughes is Assistant Director (Community Services) with Southside Partnership in Lambeth. Her background is in service management and development, and she has worked in various service settings for people with learning difficulties and those with mental health difficulties.

Steve Hurry is coordinator of a community-based day service initiative for a housing association in East Sussex, and a member of the association's training team.

Helen Jeffery is a student in social work at Bristol University. She has previously held community care posts working with people with learning difficulties from long term psychiatric hospitals, and people with learning difficulties and challenging behaviour.

Aideen Jones is Care Service Manager for a housing association in Brighton and Hove, managing a day and residential service. She spent 15 years working with young people with emotional and behavioural difficulties, and has a particular interest in training.

Jayne Kilgallen is Deputy Care Group Director, managing a supported housing service for people with learning difficulty or mental health needs. She is also manager of an Employment and Day Activities Service.

Penelope Ledger is Senior Employment Worker with Jobwise Supported Employment, giving people with learning difficulties on-the-job training and support in paid employment. She has previously worked in day services, staffed housing and social work training

Barbara Ogden is Superintendent Physiotherapist with King's Health Care Team, a multi-disciplinary health care team which provides assessment advice and clinical intervention to adults with learning difficulties, their relatives, carers and care staff.

Siobhan O'Rourke worked as a care assistant before training as a RNMH at a large mental handicap hospital, then working in various hospital and community settings. She now works with Charter Housing in South Wales, providing a community based staffed housing service for people with learning difficulties.

Jill Shepherd is Tutor and Staff Training Coordinator for a housing association in Brighton, Hove and Seaford. Her work includes training for managers and home care support staff, and developing independence skills with people with learning disabilities.

Anthea Sperlinger is Top Grade Clinical Psychologist for Services for People with Learning Disabilities, in the London Borough of Tower Hamlets.

Zenia Wainwright-Melnyk is a free-lance trainer in the field of learning disabilities, working to empower and equip direct care workers with skills to provide a quality service.

Kathy West is Coordinator of Camberwell Advocacy Office, which recruits and supports advocates in the London Borough of Southwark, provides direct advocacy for people with learning disabilities, and promotes the development of local self-advocacy groups.

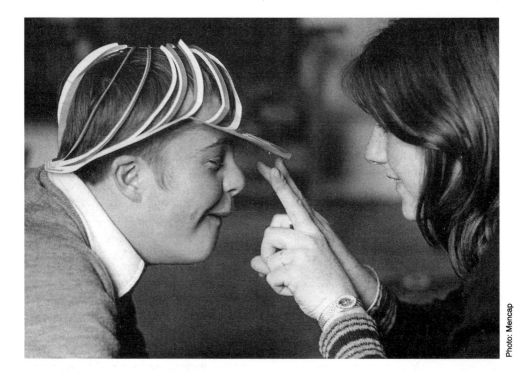

Foreword

*by Professor Sheila Hollins, Head of Division of Psychiatry of Disability,
St George's Hospital Medical School, London*

Everyone who works with people with learning disabilities, whatever their experience or aptitude, will learn an immense amount from this readable and informative book. The authors are all experienced practitioners and have adopted a practical, down-to-earth approach. All aspects of people's physical, social and emotional care are covered. The context of care is explored, several ordinary life issues are developed and many special areas such as sexuality and difficult, challenging behaviour are explained.

This will be an invaluable handbook for all staff working in residential settings. Every home should have one on its bookshelf, readily available for staff to refer to. Home leaders or officers in charge will find it an invaluable help for training and refreshing staff. For example, new staff would benefit from reading the book during their induction period, and then discussing what they have read with other staff.

Congratulations to editors and publisher for recognising the need for such a book, and masterminding it so successfully.

Introduction

Hilary Brown

This book has been designed as a practical resource for care workers in services for people with learning disabilities, in day, residential and community settings. Some of you may be called care assistants, support workers, residential social workers, nursing auxiliaries, instructors, care workers, and so on depending on what exactly you do and in what setting. We hope that the book will also prove a useful resource to people who have had training already, as it describes some new ways of delivering care to people with learning disabilities.

The people with whom you work are also referred to differently, sometimes called people with learning difficulties, or people with mental handicaps. Some people are a bit sceptical about such changes and about the one-up-man-ship which goes with getting the jargon exactly right. (Some parents of people with learning disabilities also feel this way as trends come and go). But there are three important reasons why the recent shift to the term **learning disabilities**, sanctioned by the government in 1991, should be made by all of us. Firstly, the term *learning* disability more accurately describes the difficulties which people have than the old fashioned term *mental handicap*, and it sets up expectations that these are people who, with the right kind and amount of help, can learn and develop. Learning *difficulties*, favoured by some people, does not discriminate people who have very specific difficulties, such as dyslexia, from those who have more general learning or intellectual disabilities.

Secondly, changing from *mental* handicap, makes clearer the distinction between people who have difficulties in learning from people who are suffering from mental health problems or emotional distress. People with learning disabilities do of course sometimes experience mental illness: they may get depressed, or sometimes have more serious psychiatric problems, but in this they are not different from other people. The general public tend to be ignorant about both mental illness and mental handicap, and often confuse their worst images of both so that they see everyone who is slightly different as " mad" or even dangerous. So it is very important to make this distinction clear.

Lastly, and most importantly, people with learning disabilities themselves say that this is what they want to be called, because it puts the "people" first and the "disability" second and makes clear that we are talking about a wide range of people with different strengths, needs, interests, circumstances, backgrounds and problems.

At the beginning

Learning disabilities are acquired before, at, or soon after birth, so that they affect the whole of a person's development. Common causes are chromosomal abnormalities, of which the most common is Downs syndrome; the effects of a viral infection or illness the mother has during pregnancy, as in rubella; or brain damage caused by trauma during birth, which sometimes causes cerebral palsy with or without learning disabilities. (If someone you work with has a clear "diagnosis" it is worth looking up the condition in a library to help you understand any special needs or difficulties).

Sometimes the cause of someone's disability cannot be accurately pinpointed; it may have been noticed only gradually as the mother or father became anxious about their child's progress. The time around diagnosis can be very painful for parents, and good professional support at that time is essential if parents are to feel confident of the help they can receive as their son or daughter grows up. If this has not been handled well in the past, you as care staff may bear the brunt of parents' distrust. So it is very important not to judge parents on little information.

You should also take careful note of any advice parents can give you about their son/daughter's care and development. There is nothing more galling for parents than to have worked out a pattern of caring for someone with a specific disability which is then ignored and undermined by staff in services.

A wide range of people

The group of people described in this book will be using services in very different ways. Some may live almost independently and be able to make choices for themselves with a bit of extra information and guidance; others will depend on family or care staff for help with almost all their daily needs, and making any kind of decision. These differences may be based on the extent of a person's learning disability; but for some the issue is not really how handicapped they are but the circumstances in which they have lived.

Many people with learning disabilities have lived most of their lives in barren and unstimulating institutions with no chance to develop ordinary skills, to learn about the tasks of daily living or the risks inherent in busy modern communities. That is why is important to start, as Anthea Sperlinger does in Chapter 1, by looking at the way services for people with learning disabilities have changed over recent years.

Many people still live in homes and hostels where everything is done for them and where they have little privacy, and even in newer services we can all sometimes get into an institutional way of thinking about the way we help people. The aim of an "ordinary life" is an important goal for everyone, no matter how severe their learning disabilities.

We also need to acknowledge the circumstances which bring people into contact with services, particularly their entry into residential care, prompted as it often is by resettlement, bereavement or family stress rather than positive planning or choice (see André Fox's Chapter 2).

Working with people in such settings is both demanding and rewarding, and Siobhan O'Rourke (Chapter 3) helps us to look at the caring relationships we form, balancing closeness with impartiality, friendship with professionalism.

But if ordinariness is the goal, this does not mean sitting back and letting people get on with it. It means varying the help and planning with which we support them, so that their lives are full and interesting. "Ordinary" life requires extraordinary work behind the scenes; Peter Ferns' chapter (4) on individual planning is therefore centrally important.

Good communication is also crucial, and Anne Clarke-Kehoe explains how to achieve it in Chapter 5. Tailoring what you say and how you say it to each person is also an important way of taking individual needs into account, as is acknowledging such handicaps as impaired sight or hearing (see Chapter 6).

Difficult or "challenging" behaviour

often arises from communication difficulties and lack of understanding about people's needs. Sheila Barrett in Chapter 7 describes how to assess each individual and plan a consistent approach, without which it is easy for hard pressed care workers to fall back on treating people as if they were naughty children.

The right kind of support

Once we are clear about these needs we can begin the process of planning to enrich people's lives and help them achieve valued social roles in the community. Chapters 8 to 12 look at the ways we can build in the right kind of support to people so that they can be involved in everyday household activities (Barrett), helped to learn new skills (Garnham Hooper), given assistance in planning a range of interesting day activities (Jones and Shepherd), supported in finding a job if they would like one and managing their benefits (Henderson, Crowhurst and Ledger) and encouraged in finding interesting leisure pursuits (Brennan). Then Peter Ferns in Chapter 13 looks at the additional support Black people with learning disabilities may need to maintain contact within their own communities and have their own culture respected.

Feeding and toileting people might seem an unglamorous part of the job, but the way in which these tasks are done says more about the service than almost anything else. Gee and Ogden (Chapter 14) explain how to offer help with physical care in a respectful and professional way. Chapter 15 on sexuality (Brown) explores the emotional aspects of giving intimate care, and some of the issues raised by sexual activities and relationships.

Chapter 16 on movement and lifting is essential reading if workers are to protect themselves from back injury and those who depend on them from unnecessary risk or declining mobility.

Getting good health care (Chapter 17, Higgs and Jeffery) is a responsibility of care workers and one which necessarily involves them in cooperation with other health care professionals, as a go-between with the doctor, the dentist, and other specialists. Care assistants are also crucially involved in putting professionals' advice into practice, following up on appointments and monitoring treatment. Dr David Brooks' chapter (18) explains the details of managing medication.

You need to know about people's rights so that you can challenge decisions made on their behalf or help them to make a complaint if they have been unfairly treated. Kathy West's chapter (19) on rights, advocacy and support shows how your service can build in safeguards and support people in standing up for themselves.

Chapter 20 on management (Kilgallen) demystifies the work your manager has to do to keep the service running, and Heather Hughes' chapter (21) on emergencies describes the procedures you should have in place to deal with the unexpected and avert most crises. Finally, Steve Hurry's chapter (22) outlines some training opportunities there are for you as you make your way in your career.

Making things happen

All the chapters assume that you will consult widely with people with learning disabilities themselves and with their parents and family members, so that your job will be a constant round of negotiating appropriate goals and making things happen for, and with, people with learning disabilities. And because "the proof of the pudding is in the eating", we hope that the people you work with benefit most from your reading of this book.

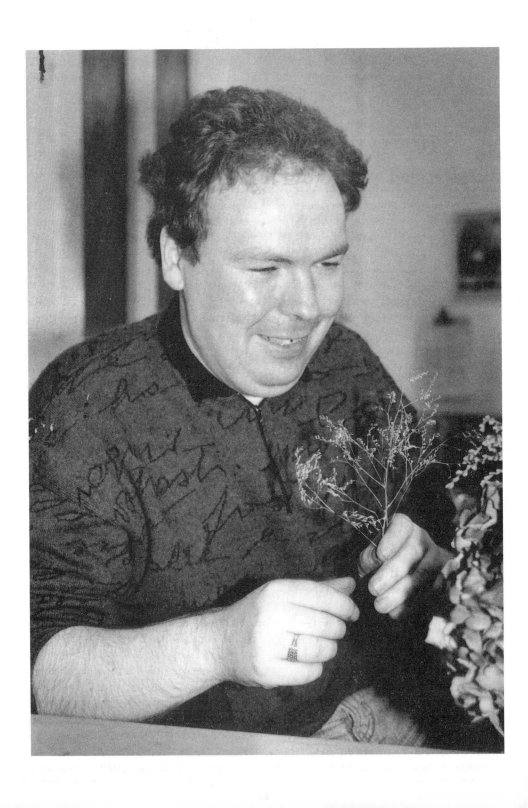

CHAPTER 1
Changing services

Anthea Sperlinger

• How services have changed, to reflect more positive attitudes to people with learning disability • Institutions • Aiming for an ordinary life • A range of services

The way in which a society views people with learning disabilities determines what kinds of services are provided for them and how they are treated by the general population. Until fairly recently, people with learning disabilities were treated as second class citizens, segregated in large institutions in rural areas or isolated within their families, and discriminated against in almost every area of their life. The last ten years have seen major changes in attitudes towards them, both as individuals and as a group, and this has been reflected in new patterns of service provision.

However, many of the negative beliefs, a lot of the buildings, and even some caring practices, remain as legacies from the past. It is therefore important to look at the history of services for people with learning disabilities and to understand people's attitudes towards them, and their families, if we are to redress the balance and to enable them to live "an ordinary life" as members of the local community.

Historical background

Attitudes towards people with learning disabilities have, until recently, been negative or devaluing. In early cultures, they were seen as being possessed by devils or being punished by God for some sin committed by themselves or their parents. During the Middle Ages, they were tortured and executed as witches or wizards, or were bought by the rich to provide amusement.

In the nineteenth century, they were separated from their families and admitted to institutions or colonies, for fear that they would have children and lead future generations of British people to become less and less able. In 1913, the Mental Deficiency Act introduced compulsory admission to institutions for people who were "mentally defective". Many people were admitted for displaying behaviour which was socially unacceptable, such as having an illegitimate child or being charged with theft.

The aims of services were to segregate people who were seen as "different" or "a nuisance" from the rest of society by placing them in large institutions in rural areas; to isolate males and females; and to protect society from people who were seen as dangerous and unacceptable. This led to the building of massive custodial warehouses which were designed to control rather than to cure.

Between 1850 and 1940, there were

widespread exhibitions of people with a learning disability for amusement and profit in freak shows[1]. These did a lot to maintain popular images of them as "exhibits" or "specimens", and to associate disability with danger.

When the National Health Service was set up in 1948, these colonies or institutions – which were built originally to segregate people with learning disabilities from the rest of society – became "hospitals" where people were "nursed" (all of their lives) and their problems were re-framed in medical terms. People with learning disabilities were seen as sick and in need of treatment, compared to other people of the same age who needed housing, education, and social care. When families could no longer cope with their son or daughter at home, they were advised to "put them away" in a "hospital" rather than being given support to enable them to continue to cope at home.

These hospitals often boasted of their "cradle to grave" services and the fact that provision for the people who lived there was "comprehensive". In fact, this meant that all services were provided on one enormous site, for up to 3,000 people of all ages. Usually, the hospital site provided laundry, catering, and cleaning services. Sick wards provided medical (even surgical) services and each hospital had its own church, chaplain and cemetery. People living in the hospital had little or no opportunity to go outside the grounds.

Institutions

Most people prefer to conduct different aspects of their life – sleeping, playing, working, for example – in different places, with different people.[2] Most of us take it for granted that we can keep different aspects of our lives relatively separate. For example, we would not expect our boss at work to sanction which people we invite for Sunday lunch, nor expect our family to be in regular contact with our work colleagues. In institutions these barriers between different spheres of life are broken down so that all aspects of life are conducted in the same place and, most importantly, under the same authority.

The central features of such total institutions in which many people with a learning disability live or have lived are:

Size: Institutions ensure that a large number of people live, work and spend their leisure time together. Activities are organised by dividing people into large batches, all of whom are treated alike and required to do the same thing, at the same time, together. People are "batched" according to their age, their sex, their disability...instead of being seen as individuals with their own unique needs, relationships and preferences.

Segregation: Institutions separate people with a learning disability from everyday community settings by providing segregated facilities and activities, so that people with learning disabilities have little or no opportunity to use ordinary community resources. Equally, the community has little opportunity to learn about them.

Location: The isolated rural location of many institutions symbolises community attitudes to people with learning disabilities. They are often surrounded by high walls and fortress-like entrances, with prominent signs announcing who lives there. They are often some distance away from shops and other local facilities, and not easily accessible by public transport.

Routines: In institutions routines tend to dominate and structure the lives of residents for the convenience of staff. For example, people are woken up at a set time, beds are made in one particular way, choices of menu are not offered, meals are served at rigidly set times and access to clean clothing is determined by the laundry service. People are helped to go to bed early so that the floors may be cleaned or the evening staff can complete their paperwork before going off duty.

The inflexibility of routines makes informality and spontaneity almost impossible and inhibits both staff and the people they support.

Privacy: It is difficult to have privacy in an institution. Your most personal activities are monitored. Toilets are often not private places, baths are rationed and may be observed, possessions are scrutinised or "vetoed" by someone in authority. Relationships with others are observed, often discussed and sometimes intercepted.

Choice: Personal choice is limited or nonexistent in institutions where residents live and share bedrooms with people staff have chosen to group together, whether or not they have anything in common or are even compatible. People do not have much choice about what to eat or wear or even how they spend their day. Many spend long periods of every day in boredom, waiting for the next routine to happen to them. On the whole, they are not involved in any of the decisions which affect their lives.

Dependence and powerlessness: Institutions encourage people to be dependent, to be incompetent, and often to perceive themselves as helpless or powerless. Many studies have shown that if we hold devaluing attitudes about people with learning disabilities and help them too much, by doing things *to* or *for* them, we reduce their confidence in their own ability and make them more dependent than they need to be. They become trapped in a "self-fulfilling prophesy" in which they are not expected to learn or to be responsible, are not given opportunities to do so, and appear not to learn or to be able to take responsibility.

Social networks: Institutions tend to ensure that people with learning disabilities are cut off from ordinary friends and acquaintances. Their social network consists of other residents, paid staff, and sometimes, immediate family members. Many lack close personal friends or have had close relationships "vetoed" or broken by re-grouping within the institution.

Traditional institutional services have

How do you rate your service?		
Size	Too big ◄——————————► Too small	
Segregation	All specialist services ◄——► Uses ordinary services	
Location	Isolated ◄——————► Right in the community	
Routines	Inflexible routines ◄——————► Flexible routines	
Privacy	No privacy ◄——————————► Privacy	
Choice	No personal choice ◄——► Involved in all decisions	
Dependence	Too dependent ◄————► Takes responsibility	
Social networks	Few friends ◄————► Large social network	

Does your service reflect old or new attitudes, institutional or community services?

denied people with a learning disability the right to have a say in their own lifestyle, and have provided them with lifestyles in which they are the passive recipients of "care". Most of us would feel outraged if someone else decided that we must move house, separate from family and friends, learn new skills and assume a certain lifestyle. Yet, for many people with learning disabilities, this is precisely what services have done.

An ordinary life

Our present goal is to see people with learning disabilities in the mainstream of life, living in ordinary houses in ordinary streets, with the same range of choices as any citizen and mixing as equals with other (and mostly) non-handicapped members of their own community.[3]

Most of us, if asked, could say what was important to us in our everyday life. Our lives revolve around our home, our family, our work, our friends and being part of our neighbourhood. Each of us chooses how to spend our leisure time, and with whom to spend this time. We find a balance between what we would like to do and what we can afford to do. We take for granted that we have a right to plan our lives and to have a say in how we lead them. It is important to us that we have chosen our lifestyle, that it has a certain value for us and that it provides us with a variety of experiences, opportunities and activities.

Traditional services for people with a learning disability rested on the assumption that *they* were not the same as you or me, and that *they* therefore did not have the same needs or rights: they were different. The principle of **normalisation**, which was developed in the 1970s, challenged this view and stated that services should start with the assumption that people with a learning disability need to have made available to them "patterns and conditions of everyday life which are as close as possible to the norms and patterns of the mainstream of society".[4]

The principle of "normalisation" contains three key elements[3]:
1. All people with learning disabilities, irrespective of their age or disabilities, have the same human rights as non-handicapped people.
2. All people, irrespective of their age or disabilities, have a right and a need to live like others in the community.
3. Service providers must recognise the individuality of people with learning disabilities, and plan services accordingly.

Normalisation is frequently misunderstood. It does not mean "making people normal". Nor does it mean that specialist services should never be used. Services based on the principle of normalisation demand that people with learning disabilities are enabled to live an ordinary life in the community with whatever support and assistance they require to do so. The five accomplishments identified by O'Brien[5] (see opposite page) provide five broad areas in which services should work to enhance the quality of people's lives.

These five related terms define the way to look at the quality of a person's life experiences. Each points to experiences which it makes sense for a person to seek more of; together they indicate a balance of experiences that make effort worthwhile. History shows that people with severe handicaps are likely to miss these ordinary positive experiences unless the people they rely on work hard to provide them.

Part of the community

Living in an ordinary house in the community does not guarantee an ordinary life. If, however, community

THE FIVE ACCOMPLISHMENTS OF NORMALISATION

Community presence: The right to take part in community life, and to live and spend leisure time with other members of the community.

Relationships: The right to experience valued relationships with non-disabled people.

Choice: The right to make choices, both large and small, in one's life. These include choices in where to live and with whom to live.

Competence: The right to learn new skills and participate in meaningful activities with whatever assistance is required.

Respect: The right to be valued and not treated as a second class citizen.

services are based on the principle of normalisation, they place the person with learning disabilities at the centre and insist that services should be designed to meet the person's real and identified needs, without imposing isolation or segregation from the local community. In addition, the community itself has to be helped to confront its own prejudices about people with learning disabilities and to help them to be genuinely integrated into community life, rather than discriminated against.

The aims of community based services

1. No person with a learning disability, however severe, is excluded from community-based services. Instead of having to prove that they are "ready" to live in the community (as in traditional services), service users are seen to have a right to live like others within the community and to be entitled to the extra help and assistance which will enable them to do so.

2. Services should be flexible and organised to meet the unique needs of each person with a learning disability in their own home, family and cultural setting. The person with a learning disability is not just expected to fit into whatever is available. Regular assessment and review of the person's needs and, where necessary, an advocate or someone to speak up on behalf of the person with a learning disability, should ensure that services respond to the person's changing needs and assist them towards the greatest possible independence.

3. People with learning disabilities should be involved as far as possible in making decisions which affect their own lives, rather than being treated as spectators while all the important decisions are made by someone else.

4. People with learning disabilities who do not live with their families, should live in ordinary houses in the community with whatever degree of staff support is appropriate to their needs. Each house should be "home" to a few people and, as they change and develop, the degree of staff support should be adjusted or withdrawn accordingly. The range of options available should vary, including for example, family placements, staffed houses, shared tenancies and independent bedsits.

5. Adults with learning disabilities who have always lived in the family home should have the same chance of moving into a home which is independent from their families as do most people. Ideally, most adults would be able to move away from home before their parents (often elderly) have reached a point of crisis (see Chapter 2). This avoids the traumatic experience which faces many people with learning disabilities, of having to move from their family environment and make a new start due to bereavement.

6. When parents or families face

How do you rate your service?	Yes	No	Sometimes
We include people with more severe disabilities			
We vary things according to individual needs and ethnic background			
We help people with learning disabilities to make choices			
We have a range of supported housing options			
We help people to live in their own homes when they become adults			
We give each family whatever support they need			
We support the person with learning disabilities' existing social networks			
We give people with learning disabilities whatever help they need to use local resources			

Think about the strengths and weaknesses of your services. Should some changes be made?

difficulties in coping with their member who has a learning disability, supportive services should be available nearby which enable the family to stay together, rather than send the person away. Each family should have support which is sensitive to their language and culture.

7. When services serve a local catchment area, they maximise the chances of maintaining someone's familiar ties and associations. Thus, services should support existing social networks which the person with learning disabilities has already established, and encourage continuity in personal relationships.

8. Living nearer community resources does not in itself guarantee greater access to them. But if people are given adequate help and support, they can have much greater access to, and use of, the amenities and resources which a typical community possesses: shops, pubs, cafes, leisure centres, libraries, adult education, etc.

9. Existing general services – ie those which are available to the rest of the community – should be used rather than separate specialist services, wherever possible. For example, general medical and dental services, chiropody, access to home helps, counselling services,etc.

10. If services which are locally based are also comprehensive, the small number of people with learning disabilities who have additional needs caused by mental illness or challenging behaviour, will have access to special help in the local community, rather than being sent away to a remote institution and separated from their family and friends. This special help may be in the form of both access to local specialist services and additional, intensive support in their own homes.

A range of services

Although the principles of "an ordinary life" have been accepted as the foundation on which services for people with a learning disability should be based, progress in establishing community based services has been slow and uneven.

• Some services are now entirely community based, while others contain a mixture of community and institutional services.

• Living in an ordinary house does not guarantee an ordinary life, and some community based services continue to segregate people with learning disabilities or to provide them with insufficient staff support. Some people with learning disabilities are isolated, bored and friendless in the community.

• Closing an institution requires complex planning and sensitive preparation to enable people with learning disabilities to move into the community. Meanwhile, services and staff face the dilemma of trying to improve the quality of people's lives within the hospital, while anticipating the upheaval of helping a large number of people to move into the community.

• Services are now provided by a combination of health, local authority, voluntary, private and housing organisations. The extent to which these agencies plan jointly and coordinate their services varies a lot from area to area.

• Community teams for People with Learning Disabilities (CTPLD) provide vital specialist support to people with learning disabilities and their families. How far they have also tried to develop access for people with learning disabilities to general services, varies widely.

Where people live and work

At home with their family: Around 40 per cent of people with a learning disability live at home with their families, and need the same sorts of support and services as do others living in the community. They may use sitting in or respite services or the support of the local CTPLD. Parents and other family members provide (unpaid) most of the support to people with a learning disability. Most services realise that family members have their own needs as individuals and that they need support in their role as carers.

Away from the family home: People with a learning disability live in institutions and in a range of local supported housing: single tenancies in ordinary houses; shared tenancies in a staffed house; living in a group home with minimal staff support; living in a local authority hostel; living with another family in a family placement. There are huge variations in the size of peoples' homes, the number of people who live together and the level of staff support which is available.

Daytime activities: Adult Training Centres or Social Education Centres are often the only resource offered to people with learning disabilities during the day. Some only attempt to "occupy" or "contain" people while others act as a resource centre which will enable people with learning disabilities gradually to use ordinary community services. Many people with learning disabilities attend adult education classes, some of which are integrated. Those who are older often prefer the lunchtime clubs and day services for elderly people in their community. There are some innovative employment initiatives which provide training, employment and continuing support for people with learning disabilities. In some parts of the country, there are successful workers' cooperatives which provide employment for people with learning disabilities. Sadly, at the other extreme, there are people who have nowhere to go during the day or who lack help to get there.

Services for people with complex needs: People with challenging behaviour, and people with additional mental health problems needing a special treatment service, are offered different services in different areas. It may be in the nearest institution, the local mental health service or in a special unit within local services for people with learning disabilities.

Sometimes this help is offered in the form of a short (respite) stay in a specialist treatment or assessment service. In other areas, help is offered by a specialist community team, who provide sensitive, intensive support in the person's home.

Advocacy

Self advocacy, in which people with learning disabilities assert their own rights, express their needs and concerns, take their own decisions and exert some control over their own lives, varies enormously from service to service. Some services are designed around Individual (or Life) Planning systems in which the person's own views, preferences and decisions are central. Other services support tenants' associations or ensure that people with learning disabilities are members of service planning and organisation committees. Quality Action Groups have been established in a number of services to ensure that users are equal stakeholders in monitoring service quality. The "People First" organisation of self advocacy groups now has branches in many parts of the country. Some of them are entirely self-directed, but many work well with the help of non-disabled advisers, who are sometimes staff.

Citizen advocacy schemes are expanding in which people with learning disabilities are personally represented in matters which affect them directly. Advocacy Alliance now has branches all over the country and several areas have citizen advocacy schemes which aim to recruit and train independent advocates for people with a learning disability.

Points to remember

1. Attitudes about people with learning disabilities determine what kind of services they are offered.
2. Historically, people with learning disabilities have been discriminated against and treated as second class citizens.
3. Institutions separate people with learning disabilities from their local community and, because of their size, location and routines, make people dependent, powerless and lacking in choice, privacy or social networks.
4. The principle of normalisation says services should be based on the assumption that people with learning disabilities should be enabled to live an ordinary life.
5. Community based services have many advantages both for people with a learning disability and for their families.
6. The five accomplishments – *Community presence, Relationships, Choice, Competence and Respect* – are important goals if we are to enhance the quality of life of the people we support.
7. The range of services for people with learning disabilities and their families varies in different parts of the country, particularly in terms of access to ordinary resources and services.
8. Self advocacy and citizen advocacy are vital if people with learning disabilities are to assert their rights, express their needs and concerns and control their own lives.

References
1. Bogdan, R. (1986) Exhibiting mentally retarded people for amusement and profit, 1850-1940, *American Journal of Mental Deficiency*, 91,2,120-6.
2. Goffman, E. (1961) *Asylums.* Now published by Penguin Books.
3. King's Fund (1980) *An Ordinary Life. Comprehensive Locally-based Residential Services for Mentally Handicapped People.* Project Paper 24. London. King's Fund.
4. Nirje, B. (1970). The Normalisation Principle - Implications and Comments. *Journal of Mental Subnormality* 31, 62 - 70.
5. O'Brien, J. (1986). A Guide to Personal Futures Planning. In Bellamy, G.G. and Wilcox, B. (Eds) *A Comprehensive Guide to the Activities Catalog: An Alternative Curriculum for Youth and Adults with Severe Disabilities*. Baltimore, Maryland. Paul H. Brookes.

CHAPTER 2

Coming into care

by André Fox

*• What brings people into residential services? • Respite care
• Leaving home • Loss and bereavement • Resettlement from hospital
• The stress of change • Careful planning to ease the transition • Maintaining
old links • Welcoming and involving families*

There are four main reasons why people with learning disabilities find themselves being cared for in a residential service. These are:
• Temporary "respite" care
• Leaving home
• Loss or bereavement
• Resettlement from hospital

It is important always to remember that change is stressful for everyone, and each person should be treated as an individual, awarded respect and given choice. If we consider our own lives, the most stressful times are in moving house and in bereavement or loss, so we need to bear in mind that some people with learning disabilities are asked to do both of these at the same time.

Respite care

One important kind of care offered to many families caring for a child or adult with disabilities is "respite" care: a temporary admission to a care establishment for anything from an evening or weekend to one or two weeks at a time. This is usually to give the parents or carers some time off from their son/daughter or relative, allowing them to go on holiday or spend time recharging their own batteries;

caring for a person with learning disabilities can be both physically and mentally demanding. Some carers use respite care more than others, which may reflect the level of support the carer requires to help the person with learning difficulties stay at home.

Respite care can be as frequent as a "week-on, week-off" system. It can be sought in an emergency or planned in advance. Emergency respite care usually comes about when a parent or carer becomes too ill to care for the person with learning difficulties, who comes into care for a set period to allow the carer time to recover. It may be that the carer has hit a sudden "low", feeling they cannot cope any more. This can be very distressing for both, so it is good practice and common sense, especially for older parents/carers, to plan ahead for respite care, in conjunction with the residential service.

A period of short visits can be arranged, leading up to an overnight stay. After a series of overnight stays the person could stay for a longer period. It may be best for the carer to stay with the person in the early stages. Care staff can help by including an activity the person likes, so that they make a link between the visit and the activity they enjoy.

Future plans

We all know that it makes sense to plan for the future, but many parents put off the decision of planning ahead for their child, because it is more than likely that this will involve coming into full-time care. This is usually a difficult decision for any parent to consider, but the question "What will happen to my daughter/son after I die?" forces the issue.

Making positive plans can help people to face the future with more confidence. Carefully planned respite care can reduce anxiety and upset for the person with learning disabilities should they need to go into residential care permanently, and enables the carer or parent to see what services are available and which would be appropriate for their child or relative.

Admission to respite care can bring some positive **advantages:**
• forming new friendships/relationships
• becoming more involved with activities which are appropriate to the person's age and interests
• providing new experiences
• gaining access to other services
• reducing future anxieties about moving
• providing an insight for the parent or carer into services available.

But there are also **problems**. Individuals or their carers may feel:
• a sense of losing their home
• fear of change and a disjointed lifestyle
• confusion and disorientation in a new environment
• loss of a certain degree of privacy, for example in sharing a room
• homesickness, missing parents, loved ones, friends, pets.

Leaving home

Often respite care will lead to a more definite decision to leave home. This can be very difficult to consider, especially if the person's difficulties are so severe that they do not understand exactly what is happening to them or why. They can become confused, upset and very anxious.

Consider your own childhood; we all have memories which we hold dear about our homes and our families and the warmth and security they afforded us. The person with learning difficulties may never have experienced an alternative to that which they already know; they may not be able to perceive what another "home" is.

For everyone, leaving home is a double-edged decision: it holds exciting prospects of independence and being responsible for ourselves without the worry and consideration of others, but we usually also have some reservations: the cost, paying the bills, shopping for ourselves, cooking for ourselves and the chores of keeping house, for example.

A lot of support

Most people with learning disabilities cannot make a decision like this without a lot of support from their carers, or a social worker or case manager who can help them balance up the *pros* and *cons*. This should not exclude or deter them from considering leaving home to live alone or in shared accommodation; but caution should be exercised so that they can move on with proper support and preparation. Every aspect must be planned for and thought through.

Leaving home because you want to, not because you have to, is something we should aim at for all people with learning disabilities, but at the moment it is the exception rather than the rule. It is much more likely that the person will move into residential services because their carers/parents cannot cope, because specialist input may be required or the individual becomes too aggressive and unmanageable.

Working with carers' and parents' feelings at the time when their child leaves home can be very difficult. There may be a sense of guilt that they can no longer cope with the care of the person, fears about the service, plus all the worry and concern of any parent whose child is about to leave home. These feelings can show in a variety of ways:

• guilt and concern
• anger, usually towards the care establishment concerned
• criticism of the level of care their son or daughter receives
• emotional upset, sometimes to the point that parents cannot visit the person
• over frequent visits to the home
• increased contact and reliance upon other professionals, the GP, social worker or Community Team for People with Learning Disabilities (CTPLD).

There is no ideal way of preparing a person with learning difficulties for leaving home. Each individual will require specific care through the whole process. But it helps if there is as much contact as possible with the home and care staff before admission, and if the person has experienced respite care regularly. One member of care staff should be "key worker" for the individual, to coordinate care and ensure good communication.

Loss and bereavement

Unfortunately people with learning disabilities are often catapulted into leaving home by the death or illness of one of their parents. This makes for a difficult and painful adjustment as they learn to live in a new setting while mourning. Often, where the individual has lived in the parental home into adulthood an unusually close relationship has developed. The twosome of husband and wife becomes a threesome of husband, wife and handicapped son or daughter, sharing household chores and leisure activities. This is very different from the relationship most adults have with their parents, especially as the parents grow older. The son or daughter may take up middle-aged pastimes such as gardening instead of activities most young people enjoy. This insular relationship makes change of any sort very upsetting. Should one of the parents die rendering the other parent unable to cope with the person with learning difficulties, there is a sudden break in the closed circle.

To bereavement is added the distress of losing their home, leaving familiar faces and places, losing contact with or responsibility for pets. If they are moved a long way from home it might feel as if they have lost everything; contact with their surviving parent may be difficult to arrange.

Grief and mourning

People with learning disabilities, like everyone else, require time to grieve after a bereavement. There are various stages to the grieving process, and these include:
(a) Loss: sorrow at the absence of the person that has died
(b) Anger and frustration: "Why did this have to happen?"
(c) Adjustment and re-adjustment: "Life must go on."

This is a natural process and everyone goes through it in their own way and at their own pace. People with learning disabilities should always be included in funerals and other mourning rituals to help them make sense of what has happened. They should be encouraged to keep pictures and reminders of the loved one they have lost.[1]

People with learning disabilities may find it very difficult to understand the concept of death, let alone know how to grieve. Some may exhibit unusual and difficult behaviours; they may have aggressive outbursts or sudden emotional disturbances. There is no set time span for grief, and if people with learning disabilities are not given support through the stages of grieving, the process can be prolonged. There is also a danger that it will not be taken into account when staff are trying to make sense of difficult behaviours. This is more likely to happen if care staff did not know the person before their bereavement.

Resettlement

Loss of a different kind may face people who are moving on, not because of their own decisions, or because their parents can no longer care for them, but because of service changes.

Since the 1970s large hospitals and hostels have been closing down in favour of smaller, more homely services in local communities. People who have lived in such hospitals may have mixed feelings and, even if to the outsider's eyes their new home looks like a great improvement, they should be encouraged to maintain links with old friends and places, to bring photos and to talk about old times. As one person said on leaving a large psychiatric hospital "I hated it there but I miss the people".[2]

Again, the transition should be planned carefully, gradually building up contacts with the new service. Attention should be paid to the way groupings are decided, and to maintaining relationships which were important to the person when they lived in the hospital.

It is easy for staff in new community services to dismiss hospitals as all bad, forgetting that the person may also have good memories over the years. Care staff in the new service must help people maintain these old links as well as enjoying new friends and opportunities.

Family links

An individual's family and friends are likely to provide the most important links with life outside the home. New contacts cannot take the place of these established relationships, especially family links.

We have already talked about the reluctance of many parents to see their son or daughter admitted into care, partly because they believe that this is the beginning of the final break of family ties. Also, it is seen as a sign of their inability to cope with their son or daughter. If they have had bad experiences of care in the past, or have misconceptions about services for people with learning disabilities, and if they have put off contact with care establishments until it became absolutely essential to use permanent residential care, all these feelings will be more acute. In this case, care staff should take pains to explain that the service is not a "last resort" but a positive, integral part of the range of community services available. They should also ensure that the family is not made to feel that the service is taking over from the family, or breaking the family up. Family members must be welcomed by staff and encouraged to stay involved with care and future plans for their son or daughter.

Where people have moved back into the community from large hospitals, parents may relive their original difficult decision to place their son or daughter there. They may feel very powerless and "fed-up" with professionals who originally "told" them to put their child in a hospital and are now "telling" them that the new ways are better. They may regret the lost years their son or daughter has spent in hospital, or feel unsure about the permanence of more informal types of care.[3]

Maintaining contact might have been difficult when visiting a hospital far away, and parents will, if made to feel welcome, find it easier keep in touch now. But you may have to re-establish links where families have slipped out of the system: informing them and welcoming contact without making them feel pressurised.

Family involvement

Parents and other family members should be encouraged from the outset to become involved in specific care procedures and training programmes for the individual. This brings dividends when the person goes home for visits, as the programmes can be continued consistently. Parents should be encouraged to discuss problems and progress with staff after home visits.

Though not essential, it is desirable that parents and carers be encouraged to meet other residents in the home, and this may help their son or daughter to integrate and feel at home with the group.

Parents' group

Some organisations have structured parents' groups or committees, like the League of Friends organisations which used to be found in the long stay hospitals. It might seem a somewhat institutional concept, but parents' groups have been found to be of great benefit to parents. They should not be restricted to fund raising but able to come together to discuss common problems and thereby alleviate stress. They may also work as a pressure group and advocate for the service within the community.

If contact stops

Many families endeavour to keep close and regular contact, visiting the service and taking the person home. But all too often, for a variety of reasons, it can become difficult for parents and family to visit and they may gradually lose touch. This causes distress both to the individual

with learning disabilities and their relative.

Services should operate an open door policy, where visitors can come and see friends or relatives at any reasonable time. You should strive to be as flexible as possible, given the commitments and activities of the home and its occupants.

Sometimes visits are very difficult, even distressing to parents or carers – for instance if their son or daughter does not acknowledge their visit. It is important that they should be able to discuss their worries with care staff after a visit such as this and that they know they can count on care staff for support and not judgment.

If visits start to drop off, care staff should try to discover the reasons, and not jump to the conclusion that families are simply not interested. Common causes are:
• lack of transport
• unemployment – reduced income to pay for transport
• increased age
• poor health
• moving house – increasing the distance from the care home
• guilt feelings or uneasiness
• emotional trauma – refusal to accept their son/daughter's admission into care.

It is important to keep records of the level of parental or family contact, how often they visit and how often the individual goes to the family home. This will make it easier to see if there are any sudden changes or a gradual reduction of contact. Care staff, or the person's key worker, should discuss this with the parents or family; or perhaps a member of the social work team can make a home visit to discuss any difficulties.

Communication

Parents, carers or relatives should meet the individual's key worker, and know this is the person they can approach to discuss issues of concern. But all care staff should be approachable; and if they cannot answer a relative's questions they should advise the parent about who is available to discuss any issues; perhaps the manager or a social worker. Parents may need help in making an appointment, and should be given all the information they need. Constant enquiries can tax the relationship between relatives and care staff; sometimes it helps to structure a parent/relative's enquiries by referring things on to a more appropriate person.

Care staff should remember that visiting relatives may have travelled a long distance at some inconvenience to themselves. They are entitled to consideration and help, and if they have any complaints or queries, staff should try to find out the nature of the enquiry, note it down and advise the parent or relative that they will get a named person to contact them by telephone to discuss their enquiry or make a future appointment if required.

Philosophies

Parents and relatives should be made aware of the philosophies of the service, including the general aims of the home and the specific goals of training programmes undertaken. Some services produce a brochure or leaflet to do this but most information can be shared face to face and any brochure used as a back-up for the care staff when they meet with the parents and relatives. Sharing some of the ideas in this book may help to ensure that staff and parents are on the same wavelength.

Points to remember

1. Change, however small, can be distressing for people with learning disabilities.
2. Respite care used positively can be a sound introduction to care services.
3. Careful planning in the use of respite care can reduce future anxiety when

coming in to permanent care is necessary.
4. Leaving home is one of the most anxious and stressful times for individuals and their families. A gradual introduction into a care service should be undertaken wherever possible.
5. Working with families is difficult but important. Relatives and parents may have problems in coming to terms with their son or daughter going into care. Parents can harbour guilt feelings about their inability to cope, and staff should give them the benefit of the doubt.
6. All possible preparations should be made before a person with learning disabilities leaves home and comes into care. Be sensitive to individual needs.
7. People with learning disabilities who have suffered bereavement and loss may express the symptoms of grief in unusual ways and their grieving may be prolonged.
8. When a person comes into care, it is vitally important to maintain family links.
9. Parents/relatives' contact should be monitored, so that if it reduces, care staff can discuss the problem and how they can help. Parents and relatives should be encouraged to form a parents' group for mutual support and advice.
10. While making the changes as smooth as possible is your aim when someone comes into care, make sure that their individual needs do not get lost.

References
1. Hollins, S and Sireling L, *The Last Taboo – Mental Handicap and Death,* video, 1985, St George's Hospital Medical School. Two booklets: *When Mum died, When Dad died,* The Sovereign Series, St George's Mental Health Library, St George's Hospital Medical School, London SW17 0RE.
2. Goldie N (1988) "I hated it there but I miss the people" – a study of ex-patients from Claybury Hospital, Polytechnic of the South Bank Dept of Social Sciences.
3. Brown H and Bailey R (1986). Working with Families. Video assisted training pack in the Bringing People Back Home series, Outset Publications (see Resources chapter)

CHAPTER 3

The caring relationship

Siobhan O'Rourke

• What does it mean to be a professional caregiver? • The nature of the relationship, and its boundaries • Planning for each individual, to involve them and give their life shape • What is a keyworker?

Most of us are so familiar with the word "care" that we never stop to think what it really means. We use the word in relation to the way we feel about family, friends, work colleagues or pets, as well as much wider issues. For example: "Susan cares about the situation in Eastern Europe"; "Mary cares about her parents"; "Margaret cares about her appearance". The word care may mean something different in each of these examples, but there is a common thread. "Care" suggests interest and concern, as contrasted with indifference or lack of concern. Caring about someone or something carries with it an implication of "taking care of" that thing or person.

How does this relate to paid caring? In the caring profession we are paid to care for, or to take care of, people. Is this different from the way we care for other people? While in many ways it is similar to personal caring, in our personal life we usually

• develop a relationship with a person
• begin to care about them, and
• begin to take care of them;

whereas in our professional life we

• begin to take care of someone

• develop a relationship with them, and
• sometimes begin to care about them.

In our personal lives, the inclination to take care of another person follows from the sense of responsibility involved in the relationship, but in our profession this responsibility starts from the fact that it is our job to provide a service involving care. This does not mean that we cannot develop a caring relationship with the people we are paid to help.

Relationships

A relationship is simply what goes on between two or more people. Relationships can be very complicated and very demanding but they are impossible to avoid. If you spend any time with other people then you have some sort of relationship with each and every person you know. We sometimes think of relationships as being very close and emotional, but not all relationships are like that. The relationship I have with my next door neighbour consists of knowing each other's names, saying hello, exchanging views about the weather, and so on. This is a relatively distant relationship compared to the one I have with my work colleagues, and not nearly as close as the one I have with my friends and family.

Obviously these descriptions are very basic, and any relationship can change. The neighbour can become a friend; a work colleague could become your partner.

Relationships can be short or long term. Short term relationships are not necessarily less meaningful or satisfying than long term ones but they involve loss which has to be planned for, and managed, by both people concerned. Staff are often advised not to develop relationships with those they care for because the relationship may only be short term, or because being close may make providing a service difficult. But relationships between staff and the people they care for are inevitable. They may or may not be positive, close, intense or satisfying, but they are part of people spending time together.

Commitment

There are responsibilities and commitments in all relationships and this applies to the care-giving relationship as well. When we are paid to do a job we have a responsibility to carry out that job to the best of our ability with the resources available to us. When that job consists of providing a care service to another person our responsibilities go further than doing good work for payment.

A professional care-giving relationship has the following characteristics:

• The client is to some extent dependent on the care staff.

• The care staff are there to meet the needs of the *client*.

• A relationship based to some extent on dependency exists between the two people.

It follows that power can play a large part in such a situation and the fact that we have power, as care staff, carries with it many responsibilities.

All social interactions take place within boundaries. These boundaries are usually based on cultural practice as well as on personal preference, for example I don't hug the bus conductor every morning and I don't address my mother as "Mrs O'Rourke" because these actions would break the usual expectations which exist in the culture I live in.

A workplace has a culture too. Some workplace cultures are formal and others are very relaxed and friendly. As care staff we often work in people's homes, whether a hospital ward, a hostel or a person's own house. This can make it difficult to know how to behave because it combines sharing with people the rhythm and flow of their domestic life (getting up, eating, bathing, housework etc), with being in the role of a paid worker. This makes boundaries extremely difficult to set.

There are no perfect answers to the question, "How close a relationship should I have with the people in my care?" but there are some guidelines. Remember:

• relationships are unavoidable

• you are paid to be a care-giver and not a friend

• you are almost always in a more powerful position in relation to clients than they are to you

• you should respect the privacy and dignity of clients

• your emotions and judgements are your own responsibility; you are not paid to love/like people, neither are you paid to tell people that you don't like them

• the relationship you develop with a client is *not* exactly the same as friendships you have in other situations because you are also in the role of a professional caregiver.

Therefore you are responsible for ensuring that the relationship is kept within professional boundaries. For example, if you see one of the people in your care a lot in your off duty time, exchange expensive presents or confide intimate secrets with each other, then you are likely to compromise the service you provide to others as well as putting yourself and them at emotional risk. You could also leave your professional reputation open to criticism, especially if your behaviour *could in any way* be perceived by the person with a learning disability, or anyone else, as being sexual.

Professional relationships can be:

• enabling

• empowering

• emotionally and practically supportive

• a learning experience

• a meaningful experience

• a satisfying experience – but also

• an experience which will sometimes be painful for both people.

For example, just when you think a person really trusts you, they bite you, or having learned to trust you the person really misses you when you go on annual leave. These painful episodes can be worked through constructively, but they could be damaging if a personal relationship without professional boundaries has developed.

Physical care

The caring role involves meeting those needs a person cannot meet for themselves, for example in the areas of personal hygiene, or assistance with cooking and cleaning. Caring for another

human being means serving them in a way that encompasses the following values:

• Safety

• Equality (just because a person is to some extent dependent does not make them inferior)

• Empowerment

• Growth

• Respect

• Dignity

Some of us may work in environments where more emphasis is placed on physical safety than on empowerment. It may not be possible to satisfy all the standards all the time but it is vital that we strive to find a balance which meets the needs and wants of the person with a learning disability. The important thing to remember is balance. Safety is essential but growth and empowerment won't take place without some carefully managed risk taking.

How do you incorporate these ideas into your daily routine?

Assisting a client with bathing is something that can be done with dignity as well as something which can provide an opportunity for empowerment. You can make a mundane event meaningful if you:

1) Know the task properly, so do it competently as well as considerately.
2) If possible give the person choice.
3) Explain what is happening as you go along.
4) Be gentle.
5) Be respectful.
6) Involve the person even if this is only through eye-contact or a smile.
7) Provide opportunities for learning and growth. For example the person might learn to let you know if they like the temperature of the water or learn to wash

their face separately, or eventually gain independence in bathing.

8) If it is safe to do so, allow the person to be totally alone in the bathroom for a while. This can be a very special time.

9) Bathtime can be made into an enjoyable and sensuous experience if perfumes, talc, soft towels, pleasant music and so on, are used at this time.

Using similar ideas you can see how easy it would be to make feeding a meal to someone a high quality experience, or to make teaching someone to dress themselves fun and interesting.

Involvement

We all learn about ourselves through messages we pick up from the people around us. Our feelings of self-worth and confidence, the belief we have that we are lovable and wanted, come from being in loving relationships.

People with a learning disability all too often receive hurtful messages: messages that they are stupid, dependent, slow, lazy, stubborn, incapable of understanding or of learning. They usually take longer to learn things, and some tasks may be beyond their potential, but that does not mean they do not feel the same range of emotions as you or I. People with a learning disability may feel hurt, rejected, insulted or patronised; they can also feel happy, loved, involved and respected.

Most of the human interaction people with a learning disability experience is with care-givers. Care-givers therefore have a responsibility to enable them to feel good about themselves. Enabling is part of our job but character judgement is not. People are sometimes described to their faces as being lazy, devious or stubborn. This does not enable the person to have a positive self image, nor does it enable the care-giver to provide a better service. Clients are entitled to our care but that does not entitle us to make personal judgements about them. Clarifying our ideas about the reasons for difficult behaviour (see Chapter 7) or poor communication (see Chapter 5) may help us to be tolerant of them even when we find them difficult.

Many care staff, myself included, were trained to be competent. At the age of eighteen I could make thirty beds, hospital style, in less than an hour and could bath ten clients in the same length of time. To take longer by offering people choice and involvement would have labelled me as lazy and a trouble-maker. The culture of many services has developed to respond to tasks rather than the needs and wants of people with a learning disability. This is probably a result of severe staff shortages as well as a different way of thinking.

Nowadays most services are aware of positive approaches to people with learning disabilities. For care staff in institutional care facilities such as hospitals or large hostels, involving people in the running of their own lives can be very difficult. However, this does not mean to say that it is impossible.

Don't despair or feel guilty if the culture you work in makes involvement difficult. Little changes can make a huge difference to a person's life. Even if you can only involve a person for ten minutes each day, that special time will be something for them to look forward to.

Of course you may be able to go a lot further than that and involve them in every aspect of their daily lives. Where I work as a community care coordinator, people with a learning disability are involved in choosing their own furniture, food, clothes and other possessions, and many of them have been involved in choosing who comes to live and work with them. They are also involved in housework, cooking, shopping and a range of leisure activities to the best of each person's ability. This did not happen overnight. Real involvement in daily activities requires careful planning (see Chapter 8 on Participation).

Planning to give life shape

The staff team at a home known as Montgomery Street wanted the service to be as homely as possible, and so there was no structure or planning from the day the service opened. A year later the people who lived there had very little social life, spent most of their free time watching videos chosen by the staff, couldn't cook, clean the house or shop independently and found it almost impossible to form their own opinions or make choices. They had frequent arguments which often led to aggression.

When structures and planning were introduced, people were involved in planning their daily routines with help from the staff. Six months later the people who live at Montgomery Street were much more confident and involved in the running of their home. They not only cooked, shopped and cleaned the house needing very little assistance, but they also helped to devise a staff rota which suited their needs, and enjoyed much more satisfying social lives. Assertiveness training and counselling as well as skills teaching contributed to the positive changes that took place for these people.

People need to be connected with the details that form everyday life. Otherwise life loses its shape and its meaning. This is related to learning and practising specific skills so as to be able to have some control over events. For example, Alex loved tea and was constantly asking staff to make some for him. He was frustrated by his dependence on others. After learning to make tea, he now makes it for himself as well as others, so it has given him some independence and status.

Participating

Involvement in the flow of life comes from participation. Many people with learning difficulties do not initiate activities, so if care staff don't create opportunities for participation their lives can be flat, dull and monotonous. Some repeatedly inquire about the rota: "Who's on tomorrow, who's on after that..." Perhaps this is related to the lack of contrasts in their lives, the only variety being the faces of the staff team. See Chapter 8 for ideas on how to involve people more.

To start you off, choose one of the people you work with:

• Plan things so that they get out to the park or the shops once a day.
• Plan time for one-to-one contact where the person is not necessarily being asked to do anything.
• Plan active times and quiet times.
• Plan teaching times and pleasure times.

But you may need to change the rota or coordinate work differently; there is no point planning a routine with someone, then finding there's no time to go to the bank or fill in the petty cash forms.

Good planning means balancing all the different things that go on in a service and making sure that all the really important things get done on time. A shift plan can help everyone to co-ordinate events.

Have a good time

In a human service things don't always work out as planned. Don't take it too seriously; remember to have a good time together with clients. If people are learning, are making choices, are smiling and laughing more and seem to be getting a kick out of life, then the plan is working. If it is a system imposed on staff and hence in turn on clients it will not result in improved quality of life.

The keyworker

Helping someone to plan their daily life will highlight areas where they may want or need skills teaching (see Chapter 9) or where they may want or need access to facilities not currently on offer to them. For example someone may want a job (see Chapter 11). In order to be able to offer effective help and support to people, it is useful to organise a keyworker system within the service.

This means that each person with learning disabilities has one member of staff allocated especially to them in order to co-ordinate the activities, services and experiences that enhance their life.

Jacky is Martin's keyworker. Her jobs include:

• Helping Martin keep in touch with his family;

• helping to order and collect his medication;

• keeping records of how well Martin is doing;

• helping him to buy new clothes;

• organising and attending Individual Programme Planning (IPP) meetings to plan things formally with Martin;

• communicating with the rest of the team to make sure that Martin receives the support he wants and needs.

The rest of the staff are involved in caring for Martin but it is Jacky who has primary responsibility for empowering Martin and making sure his voice is heard.

Being a keyworker means advocating for the person with a learning disability. Advocating means speaking on behalf of another person and making sure you say what you think he or she wants you to say. It is not good enough for Jacky to say "Martin wants more exercise" if Martin has made an informed choice not to take any more exercise. Jacky could say that she feels he needs more exercise, but that is a different thing from claiming to speak *for* someone.

So naturally, in order to speak for someone, you must get to know them and find out what *they* want. You have to be really careful not to mix up what you want for the person and what the person really wants for themselves. For example, Jeremy, Keith's keyworker, thought that Keith would really enjoy literacy classes (evenings at the local school).

Jeremy believed it would empower Keith and increase his self-esteem and independence. Jeremy was very enthusiastic about it, and arranged for Keith to attend the classes. He accompanied Keith to the first few classes but Keith then refused to continue. After much discussion, it emerged that Keith really wanted to go to greyhound racing every Sunday. This was less convenient for the staff than a local evening class so it was very difficult for Jeremy to advocate for it – but he did.

So as a good keyworker you should:

• Get to know the person.

• Find out what *they* want you to say for them.

• Be careful not to put your own ideas forward instead of representing the person with learning disabilities.

• Be aware that the person may ask for something that makes demands on staff.

Points to remember

1. **Relationships:** keep within professional boundaries.

2. **Physical care:** consider safety, equality, empowerment, dignity, respect, growth.

3. **Involvement/Participation:** doesn't actually take up more time than excluding people from everyday tasks.

4. **Planning:** necessary but keep it flexible.

5. **Keyworking:** enables people with learning disability to set and achieve *their* goals.

CHAPTER 4
Individual planning

Peter Ferns

-

• Defining oppression and devaluation • Understanding the experiences of people with learning disabilities • Promoting equality and socially valued roles • The importance of person-centred planning • Six steps for producing an Individual Plan

Many care services have developed into large organisations, and like other large organisations they have a great number of rules and regulations and do not deal with people as individuals very easily. The difference between care organisations and other types of organisations is that they deal with large numbers of vulnerable, disadvantaged and less powerful people in society.

It would be easy to ignore the wishes and interests of these groups of people, so it is even more important that a care organisation protects the rights of individuals through its ways of working and the systems it operates.

Individual Planning is one important way of working that can ensure that care services really do meet the needs and wants of people with learning disabilities. It is a way of planning the services which are delivered to the person and their family, which puts the individual, their family and friends at the centre of the whole process. Individual Planning aims to make sure that people who use services:

• have valued experiences in the community;

• are helped to discover a desirable personal future;

• feel more in control over their own lives;

• are protected from discrimination.

• have their links with family, friends and community strengthened.

• have their needs met in a way that strengthens communities.

Oppression and devaluation

Oppression is:

• ways of thinking, prejudiced attitudes and beliefs about groups of people in society that deny them their individuality and stereotype them;

• abuse of power, where power and control over their own lives is taken away from people and their influence in society is reduced;

• institutional discrimination from organisations in society, resulting in unfair treatment, reduced life opportunities and social injustice for certain groups of people.[1]

Devaluation is:

• seeing people as inferior because of differences in appearance and behaviour. This negative perception has a variety of consequences for the devalued person, significantly restricting their life opportunities and experiences.

What happens to people

Many people with learning disabilities will have experienced both oppression and devaluation in their lives. **Diagram 1** opposite outlines how this process happens to an individual, and the way traditional services have responded.

These devaluing and oppressive experiences can be changed for people with learning disabilities, and care services can play a leading role in this positive change. **Diagram 2** on page 34 shows how the negative cycle of experiences can be replaced with a positive cycle of equality and the development of socially valued roles in the community.

Person-centred planning

Be clear about the influence and power of services in individuals' lives

Services have a big effect on the lives of people who depend on them, over a long period of time, in the following areas :

• Places – *where* the person lives, learns, works and plays.

• Activities – *what* the person does in their daily life.

• People – *who* the person gets to know.

• Times – *when* the person does things in their daily life.

• Reputation – *how* people see themselves as well as how others see them.

Respect individuality and personal differences

Person-centred planning avoids "block" treatment of people and provides a more individualised service. It also counteracts the tendency of services to define people's needs in terms of the services available and to fit people to services rather than the other way around. The result is a more personal service that is less bureaucratic and mechanical.

Empowering individuals

Person-centred planning helps us to focus on the individual as a person and not a collection of problems. This approach will ensure that individuals' needs are seen as the most important factor, not the service's needs. Planning in this way will help to create a more equal power relationship between the worker and the individual and it will be less likely that the individual will be blamed for any failure of the service.

Making effective use of services

The service is given help to focus on specific actions and does not waste time and resources doing less effective things with the individual. The roles of service workers are clearer and their efforts are better coordinated. Planning helps to structure the work with individuals who may have complex needs, making the tasks of service delivery more manageable for workers. It will also help workers and people with learning disabilities to map their achievements more easily.

Increasing accountability to individuals and their families

A plan makes it clearer to individuals and their families about what the service is offering to them. It increases accountability to individuals by producing a written commitment which can then be monitored and reviewed.

Supporting individuals to discover a desirable personal future

Individual plans help people with learning disabilities, families and carers to make informed decisions about what are the most important needs to meet now for individuals. Plans enable services to create more opportunities for valued experiences in the community for people with learning disabilities, and generate new options for them. Plans are a valuable way of enabling

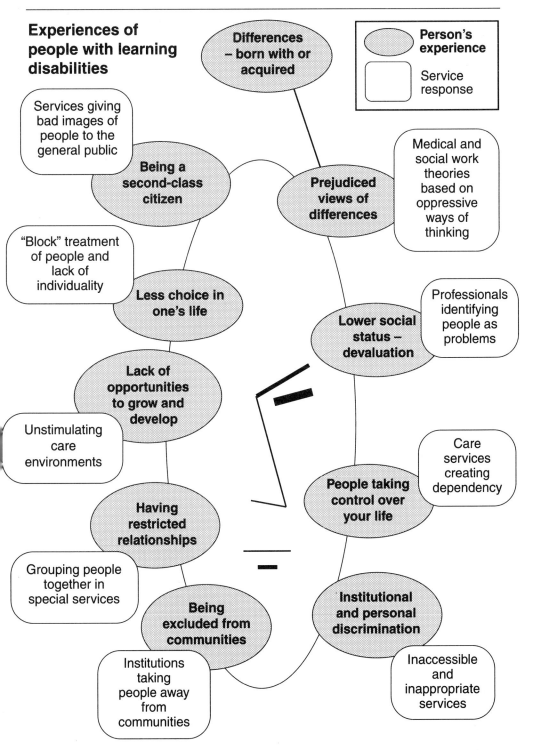

Experiences of people with learning disabilities

Differences – born with or acquired

Person's experience

Service response

Services giving bad images of people to the general public

Being a second-class citizen

Prejudiced views of differences

Medical and social work theories based on oppressive ways of thinking

"Block" treatment of people and lack of individuality

Less choice in one's life

Lower social status – devaluation

Professionals identifying people as problems

Lack of opportunities to grow and develop

Unstimulating care environments

Care services creating dependency

People taking control over your life

Having restricted relationships

Grouping people together in special services

Being excluded from communities

Institutional and personal discrimination

Institutions taking people away from communities

Inaccessible and inappropriate services

Diagram 1. The experiences of people with learning disabilities.

Promoting equality and socially valued roles

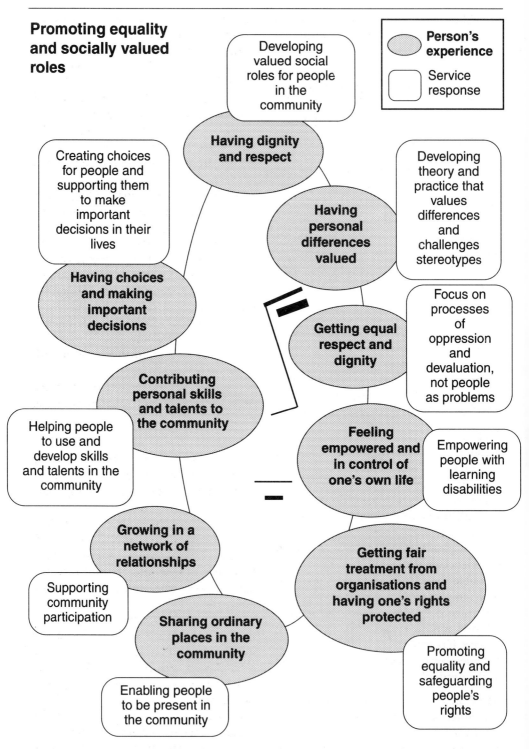

Diagram 2. Promoting equality and socially valued roles.

individuals and carers to move towards achieving a desirable personal future for the individual[2].

Making an Individual Plan

STEP 1. Setting up the Individual Planning process.

What to do:

• Find out how the individual communicates and think about the consequences for your work.

• Find out whether the individual has or needs an advocate, or someone who can represent their interests.

• Get permission from the individual or their advocate to contact family, friends and carers.

• Explain to individuals or advocates the purpose and process of planning, giving some idea of the timescale involved.

• Negotiate the ground rules for the work.

• Agree how the information will remain confidential and who will have access to it.

• Talk through any individual anxieties.

Pointers:

• Establish a relationship of trust with individuals and their families.

• Be clear with individuals and families about your role and responsibilities: you can tell them you are there to collect information and support the individual to make a plan to help them have valued experiences in the community.

• Enable the individual to have as much power as possible in decision making.

• Involve individual, family, advocates, friends and carers in the planning process, if possible.

• Remember that services can never meet *all* the needs of individuals.

STEP 2. Getting to know the person and collecting information.

What to do:

• Communicate directly with the individual as well as you can (use an interpreter if necessary).

• Spend time with the individual at different times in their day, listening and observing.

• Contact family, friends and carers and explain the purpose of planning.

• Share a meal with the person in the service setting or family home.

• Visit the person's work or education setting.

• Attend and observe any meetings where decisions are being made about the person, for example staff meetings.

• Observe any outside recreation or organised leisure activity at least once.

• Work out a weekly schedule for the person to see where they spend most of their time.

• Discuss the services being offered with the individual and families.

• Get access to records and liaise with other service providers.

• Check out information gained with the individual and family, including going through files.

Pointers:

• Always spend most time with the individual, communicating and listening – he or she is your first and most important source of information.

• Get to know the person first, before trying to get more detailed or second-hand information from files or such like.

• Be sure to take into account race and cultural issues when working with a black individual.

• Think about the kinds of stereotypes that might be put on to the person because of their race, gender or sexuality.

• Think about the person's differences in a positive way; don't see them just as problems.

• Don't make assumptions that the person's situation will never change.

• Don't see anyone as too disabled to

benefit from improved life situations.

• Don't focus on the disability and miss seeing the person.

• Talk to the most important people in the person's life.

• Observe how other people behave when they are with the person.

• Don't rely too heavily on past records. Find out about the person now.

• Use records initially only to get contacts and basic health information. Don't review them in depth until later, when there has been greater contact with the person and others.

• Decide how to record your information, bearing in mind that you will need to share the information with individuals and families. Use a variety of ways of recording such as tape, video and photos.

STEP 3. Making a personal profile.

There are many ways in which the information about the person can be put together and one way is set out below. The most important things about this information are: whether it gives a picture of the whole person, and how useful it is in helping the individual to have more valued experiences now and work out a desirable future.

Personal qualities

The aim of this part of the profile is to get an idea of the person as a unique individual with strengths and talents – to get to know what the person is like in terms of their interests, preferences, appearance and personality. Remember that the person may well have had their interests and ideas ignored for a long time.

Useful questions to have in your head:
– *What is the race, gender and sexuality of the person?*
– *How has the person dealt with oppression and discrimination?*
– *What does the person like doing most?*
– *What does the person least like doing?*

Physical health care needs

This section addresses the physical well-being of the person and highlights any drugs or any other medical treatment required by the person. It also looks at the use of the person's GP, their dental care, screening and use of health care resources. The way in which a person's physical health affects their daily care is examined in relation to feeding, bathing, toileting, lifting and nutrition.

Useful questions :
– *In what ways does the person's disability complicate their life?*
– *Are the person and their carers aware of the person's health care needs?*
– *How are the person's cultural and religious needs being catered for in their physical care, eg skin and hair care for African-Caribbean people.*

Mobility issues

The ability of the person to physically get around the community should be investigated here. Access to community transport, aids to mobility, training for travel are all factors in physical mobility.

Useful questions:
– *What kind of support does the person require to get around the community?*

Communication

It is important to look at the ways the individual communicates with others, particularly if they have no speech, or have sensory impairments. Black and minority ethnic individuals may have other language needs if English is not their first language. Signing, the use of "lip speaking" and large print for visually impaired people should all be considered. Behaviour is also an important form of communication that should not be overlooked, and the best people to consult may be the person's family or long term carers.

Useful questions:
– *What supports, aids or people can enable direct communication with the person?*

Social networks

Relationships with the natural family at present and in the past need to be asked about. Personal relationships with friends and those people who are special to the person should be identified. Particular attention should be paid to relationships in the community, outside services.

Useful questions :
– *Which people have the most power and influence in the person's life?*
– *Who are the person's friends and what sort of things does the person do with them?*
– *If the person is black or from a minority ethnic group, do they have friends who are from their own racial and cultural background? If they have no social contacts with black people, why is this?*
– *What relationships does the person have with people who do not use services or work in services?*

Past

Involvement with family, carers, friends, lovers would all be important experiences to identify. Significant events in the person's life, important changes the person has been through, the good times and the bad times should be recorded. Of course, it would be ideal if the person were supported to write their own life story. A variety of methods could be used, not just writing. Pictures, films, video, visiting old places and familiar people from the past could form a valuable activity for the person, if they wished. Where the person has lived and where they were educated are also important areas to explore.

Useful questions:
– *What have their experiences prepared the person for?*
– *Has the person missed out on any important*
common life experiences?
– *What labels or stereotypes have been attached to the person by care professionals, and what have been the effects of these labels?*
– *What has been the significance of the person's race, gender and sexuality in their life?*
– *How was the person involved with care services in the past and how good an experience was it?*

Present situation

The focus here should be on what life is like now for the person:
• where the person spends most time and what happens in the various places where they spend time;
• the kind of roles the person has in the community and the way these roles may be changing;
• the major changes happening in the person's life at present and how they are coping with them;
• the person's financial situation and their work prospects;
• the current labels or stereotypes the person is experiencing, and their consequences for the person. If there are any negative labels about a person's behaviour, try and find out exactly what this behaviour is, how frequently it happens, under what conditions and what follows the behaviour (see Chapter 7).
• Consider what are the major problems in living facing the person, how they are dealing with them, and what has been of most practical help.

Useful questions:
– *Where and with whom does the person spend most time?*
– *What does the person enjoy doing most/least?*
– *What are the person's greatest skills and most positive attributes, and which of them are wanted or needed by others?*
– *What links with the community does the person have? If the person is black, what links with black communities do they have?*
– *What types and levels of support does the*

person require?
– What future does the person have to look forward to and what are his/her dreams and aspirations?

STEP 4. Identifying needs and wants.
What to do:
• Use the five Valued Experiences, set out below with some useful questions to think about when you work with individuals, advocates and families on this issue. Examine the person's current experiences under each of the headings , and go on to identify a possible future improvement.

SHARING ORDINARY PLACES
What kind of community settings does the person go to (not care services)?

How does the person go into the community, in a large group or on their own, with support etc?

What kind of transport does the person make use of?

Does the person make use of community facilities in a way that encourages meeting local people?

What kind of information does the person have about what's happening in the local community?

Does the person have any problems in using community facilities?

What can be done to enable the person to use community facilities more: eg increased skills, more assistance, mobility aids, negotiating changes in the facility, changing what the service does?

GROWING IN RELATIONSHIPS
What relationships does the person have with people who are not connected to the service setting?

Does a black or minority ethnic person have contact with people from similar racial or cultural backgrounds?

Does the person have any friends or allies who could advocate for them, if they need an advocate?

What contact does the person have with their existing family network?

Whom does the person approach to talk about their personal problems and worries, or go to for comfort?

How does the person deal with any anxieties they may have about meeting new people? What skills does the person have in this area?

CONTRIBUTING TO THE COMMUNITY
Does the person belong to any community groups such as churches, temples, mosques, community centres, clubs, black groups, women's groups, lesbian and gay groups, sports clubs, tenants' associations etc?

Does the person help anyone else in the community?

Has the person learned new skills in the past year? How have they learned these new skills?

What skills could help the person most in having valued experiences?

What skills does the person use to deal with their life problems now?

What educational opportunities does the person have?

MAKING CHOICES
What small everyday choices and major decisions does the person make in their life? Who does make these decisions if it is not the person?

Do the options available to the person reflect and strengthen their cultural preferences (food, clothes, music etc)?

How is the person consulted about things that affect them? Do people around the person act on their views and wishes?

How aware is the person of their civil rights? What support does the person get in exercising these rights, such as voting, making complaints about racial or sexual harassment?

How is the person involved in making decisions about who cares for them and in the hiring of care staff?

What kind of sexual identity does the

person have and how do they choose to express their sexuality?

How does the person respond to taking risks, trying out new things and coping with occasional failure?

What skills does the person use to deal with oppression?

What skills in assertiveness does the person have?

How does the person speak out for themself or stand up for their rights?

HAVING DIGNITY AND RESPECT

Does the person have as much privacy in their life as any ordinary citizen?

Does the person project a positive image in the community in terms of appearance, behaviour and dress?

Does the person get respect for their cultural preferences in personal care, food, appearance, dress and spiritual needs?

How aware is the person of their rights to challenge the quality of care they are receiving?

What valued community roles does the person fulfil?

What community roles would best enable the person to express their talents and skills?

Are there any health problems affecting the person's growth and development? How can these problems be dealt with, with least disruption to the person's everyday life?

What to do

• Focus on a few needs and wants arising from the Valued Experiences exercise and find out what is most preferred by the individual, advocate and family.

• Decide on what changes would make the biggest impact on the person's life experiences now.

• If there are differences of opinion, work out why and make a plan to deal the situation.

• Be clear about any barriers to valued experiences for the person. Work out ways

these barriers could be removed.

• Make a summary of a desirable future for the person, and share it with everyone involved in the planning process.

Pointers:

• Don't be quick to dismiss the person's ambitions and aspirations as "unrealistic". See what it would take to achieve them.

• Focus on the person's needs first without thinking about service constraints, or else there will be a tendency to fit the person's need into existing services.

• Increase the person's control of the immediate environment, choice of activities and people assisting him/her.

STEP 5. Working out ways to meet needs and wants.

What to do:

• Gather information about the local community – people and places, facilities and cultures.

• Make as many personal contacts as possible with local people who may be a useful resource in linking the person more to the community.

• Make suggestions, encourage and help community facilities to adapt their service to meet the needs of the person.

• Communicate clearly the kind of help that facilities and people can offer the person.

• Work out what the person can offer to others in these facilities.

• Enable the person to feel comfortable in using facilities by introducing them personally and giving information about the person's needs.

Pointers:

• Avoid jargon and negative language about the person with learning disabilities when giving advice and information to people in the community facilities.

• Work to strengthen and educate community facilities and services, thereby making community resources more accessible to people with disabilities in the future.

• Use mainstream resources as much as possible to enable the person to feel they are an ordinary member of the community, but don't let them go without specialist services when these are in their interests and might open up other ordinary opportunities in their wake. For example a "special" and thorough hearing assessment may be well worth it if the person is able to make relationships more easily as a result of it. In this model specialist services should be seen as a means and not an end.

STEP 6. Making an agreement about the Individual Plan.

What to do:

• Write a summary of the desirable future that is seen for the person.

• Identify and write down the supports which the person will receive – people, group support from peers, aids and equipment.

• Detail the goals that have been decided upon, making sure that they are clear, precise and understandable to the person or advocate.

• Detail what the service will provide over a specified time.

• Write down what the person, advocate and family can do if they are not happy with the way the plan is being put into practice.

• Agree a date to review the plan with all the people involved in putting it together.

Pointers:

• Check that the plan does not see the person's needs just in terms of existing services.

• Always ask yourself whose needs are being met by the plan. Is it really the person's needs or is it the service's or family's needs?

Points to remember

1. Many people with learning disabilities will have experienced oppression and devaluation in their lives.

2. Care services can play a leading role in positive change for people with learning disabilities if they aim to promote equality and develop socially valued roles for individuals.

3. Person-centred planning is important because:

• services have great influence and power in the lives of people who use them over a long period of time;

• it helps services to respect individuality and personal differences;

• it empowers individuals;

• it leads to more effective use of services;

• it increases accountability to individuals and their families;

• it supports individuals to discover a desirable personal future.

4. There are six steps for producing an Individual Plan:

• Setting up the process

• Getting to know the person and collecting information

• Making a personal profile

• Identifying needs and wants (including the Valued Experiences)

• Working out ways to meet needs/ wants

• Agreement about the Individual Plan.

References and further reading

1. Adapted from "Framework for the Future" by P. Ferns, K. Kurowski, L. Colledge & P. Wakeford (unpublished).

2. Many of these ideas were developed through co-training with Tim Stainton.

Brost M. & Johnson T.Z. (1982) "Getting to Know You – One Approach to Service Assessment and Planning for Individuals with Disabilities" published by Madison WI, Wisconsin Coalition for Advocacy.

O'Brien J. & Lyle C. (1987) "Framework for Accomplishment". Lithonia Ga: Responsive Systems Associates.

CHAPTER 5
Towards effective communication

Anne Clarke Kehoe

• What is communication? • How can we encourage people to communicate? • Listening and responding • What to say and how to say it • Gestures and other clues • The special problems of impaired sight and hearing – what to look out for and how to help

Communication is a highly complex skill. Nevertheless most of us master it by the time we are five years old, usually with little effort.

We often describe someone's communication skills in terms of how well they can express themselves in either words or signs. But it is essential to remember that communication is a two way process. Before someone can begin to send messages with meaning, they have to have developed skills and strategies for understanding the world around them.

We are all highly skilled communicators (most of us know over 14,000 words), and because communication is so easy for us, we take it very much for granted. We therefore need to remind ourselves of what our lives would be like if we could not communicate effectively.

For instance, have you ever been in a situation where you cannot understand what is being said? Maybe you are in a foreign country. How do you feel?

• Isolated   • Confused
• Angry   • Inadequate
• Helpless   • Ignored
• Paranoid (are they talking about me?)

Have you ever experienced the frustration of trying to tell someone something, and they just cannot understand what you mean? How do you feel?

• Frustrated   • Inadequate
• Angry   • Like giving up

A person with very restricted communication skills may be experiencing these feelings for much of the time.

So it is not surprising that many people with learning disabilities either give up communicating, and are then described as withdrawn, uncooperative or even lazy, or develop behaviours which are regarded as difficult or challenging. These may be simply a response to the frustration of having limited communication skills, or the challenging behaviour may be the only effective way the person has of making sure they are "listened to".

Communication is a central factor in almost everything we do in life. If for any reason we cannot communicate effectively, it is a barrier to:

• making relationships;
• learning new skills;
• having our needs met;

- making choices;
- projecting our own identity and personality;
- taking part in family, community, leisure pursuits;
- making sense of the world.

For these reasons, developing a person's communication skills should be a priority, and will almost certainly be done most effectively in their everyday environment, with care staff and family members they are familiar with.

Motivation

The two most important principles which underlie successful communication are:

1. If someone sees communication as ENJOYABLE, they will want to use it, and develop it.

If they see it as boring, very hard work, they get ignored, or are not given enough time, they may give up trying altogether.

2. We must create opportunities for people to experience SUCCESS at communicating.

If they repeatedly fail, or are ignored, they will not be motivated to keep trying, or learn new skills.

For some people with learning disabilities, one of the biggest obstacles to them developing spontaneous communication is a lack of motivation. This may have developed because when they do signal that they want something no one takes any notice, or their request is misunderstood or refused.

By trying to ensure that their communication is successful as often as possible, and is enjoyable, we are much more likely to create some motivation.

How much does the person understand?
Many people appear to understand much more of what is said to them than they actually do. We usually assume they understand because they respond appropriately when spoken to, at least some of the time. However, in reality, many have limited ability to understand spoken messages, and have developed strategies for trying to make sense of their world through non verbal, situational clues, for example a point or gesture (that we may not even realise we are giving), the behaviour of another person, a well known routine, etc.

It is very easy for us to be misled into thinking someone must have responded because they understood what was said. Sometimes it seems as if the sentence we said was so complicated, a non verbal clue could not possibly have given enough information. But could it?

Take these examples:

1. "Come on Frank, put your coat on quickly, it's time to go shopping"

When Frank puts his coat on, and goes to wait by the front door, we naturally assume he has understood what we have asked him to do, and where he is going.

However, in reality, he may be just responding to the fact that you pointed towards the coat cupboard when you spoke, and he knows that whenever you put a coat on, you must be about to go out.

2. "Sue, could you take your plate out to the kitchen and give it to Pam"

Sue responds exactly as requested. Again, we are reinforced into thinking she must understand what is said to her.

In reality, she responds because you have just asked another person to do the same task, and when you speak to Sue, because she has finished her dinner, she assumes you are asking the same thing. When she gets to the kitchen, Pam is the only person there, so Sue gives her the plate.

We need to find out how much of someone's ability to respond is because they understand what is said to them, and how much their response is due to other clues. It is important to do this for the following reasons:

1. To highlight the need to adjust the quantity and quality of our input.

2. To explain why bizarre, inappropriate or even challenging behaviour may occur.

3. To indicate when someone would benefit from additional, non verbal clues eg: signs, pictures, objects or symbols, to help them interpret messages..

If we think someone is responding because they understand what is said to them, our expectations will be too high. When sometimes they fail to respond, or respond inappropriately, the natural consequence is for us to interpret this as laziness, disobedience, sulking, deliberate wind up, etc. In reality, the non verbal or situational clues that the person needs may just not be present. In this situation they may either feel too unsure to respond at all, or act on whatever clues are present, but these lead them to interpret the message incorrectly, and therefore respond inappropriately.

Assessment

A speech therapist can carry out a formal assessment of a person's ability to understand spoken language by various methods including the Derbyshire Language Scheme. But there are informal ways which can be used in the person's home or workplace to try and determine whether they are responding to spoken information, or relying upon non verbal or situational clues.

One way of testing is to make a list of phrases which you think the person understands. Discuss with other people who know the person in the appropriate context, what other clues could be

operating. Then test out the phrase, in a situation when it would naturally occur, but with all clues removed.

For example
Phrase: Please go and get your slippers
Possible non verbal clues: gesture – point, head nod etc; time of day, eg bedtime; he has just taken his shoes off; he has just come in from outside; someone else just went to get their slippers, etc.
Create a test situation when someone has been in room for a while, with his shoes on, at a time when he would not normally remove them. No one else should have just got their slippers. Say the sentence to him, and make sure NO gestures are used.

If there is no or limited response, try introducing a clue, eg: point towards the slippers. This will give you an idea whether this is the real thing which makes him understand.

Another method is to try just using gesture with no speech, or speech which is meaningless in that situation.

For example, point at the slippers and say: "What a lot of snow we had today."

If the person responds by getting his slippers, or walking to them, it indicates that the non verbal, situational clues are the ones he relies upon most to interpret his world.

This can be true of people who score on formal assessments as being able to understand some of what is said to them. When they are out of the test situation, and back at home or work in a noisy environment with its many distractions, verbal messages may not be as easy to interpret as they were in a quiet test situation.

Understanding key words

There are undoubtedly many people with learning disabilities for whom the spoken word is virtually meaningless.

There are also many who are at the stage of being able to understand just one or two key, familiar words in any one sentence said to them.

While this is undoubtedly an advantage for the person, it can lead to:

1. A greater likelihood of families and care staff thinking that the person understands almost everything they say.
2. An increase in the chances of the person wrongly interpreting something that is said to them.

This can lead either to the person being told off for responding inappropriately , or them becoming very disappointed, upset or even angry because some expectations they have formed have not materialised.

For example, Jennifer overhears two staff members talking:

"Hi Pam, did you go swimming last night?"

Perhaps she only understands one word in the sentence – "swimming". She does not realise that the message is not meant for her, and begins to feel excited at the prospect of going swimming.

Care staff cannot understand why Jennifer is excited, and keeps using the Makaton sign for swimming.

Eventually they become irritated with her, and tell her off. She becomes angry and hits a member of staff.

The care staff are unaware of Jennifer's limitations and therefore cannot see how the situation could have arisen. Also, the explanations which they start off by giving, for example –

"It's not your swimming day today"

"What's the matter with you, you know you don't go swimming on Tuesday"

– are too complex. Jennifer will again only understand the key word "swimming" which reinforces her expectations.

When the swimming doesn't happen, or she is restrained from going to the minibus, she feels let down, or may even interpret it as a punishment for no apparent reason. Challenging behaviour may be the result.

Even if we cannot accurately determine how much a person understands, it is a good idea always to reinforce your spoken message with gestures, pictures etc. If a person does not need the help of extra clues, they will just ignore them.

What you say, and how

• Make sure the person knows that the message is meant for them. Make sure you have their attention, and speak/sign/show an object or picture within their visual field.

• Try to use consistent vocabulary. Many people will be confused if different names are given to the same item – coat, jacket, anorak, windcheater, for example.

• Use short, straightforward phrases, which are in adult style but do not contain any unnecessary extra information.

For example: "Paul, get your coat" (four words) is better than "Paul, can you hurry up and get your coat on, the minibus will be here soon" (sixteen words).

We tend to use longer messages like this, but they are much more likely to be misinterpreted. We are also more likely to lose the person's attention.

• Break down long multi-message phrases into separate messages. This not only makes it easier for the person to understand, but also means that you may have several opportunities to say "Well done" rather than becoming exasperated because the person has responded inappropriately. For example: "Mary, can you find your swimming things and put your coat on, then get into the car" – could become:

"Mary, get your swimming things...Well done...Now put your coat on...Well done...

Now get in the car...Great."

• Try to avoid using complex language structures:

People with severe learning disabilities have particular difficulties understanding time concepts, so words like *tomorrow, this afternoon, at three o'clock, later, soon* are often meaningless, which is why a person may keep returning to ask "is it time for swimming" even though we have told them swimming is this afternoon.

Negative words, those which mean no – *not, can't, isn't, wont, haven't, don't* – are also very difficult for some people to understand. If they cannot understand these words, they will hear the message as if it is going to happen. This could have far reaching consequences. For example, if you say, "You are not going swimming this afternoon" someone who cannot understand negative concepts will receive the message, "You are going swimming this afternoon".

They may become very frustrated and even angry if anyone tries to stop them going. They will certainly be disappointed.

In these situations, try to avoid using negative words, and whenever possible, talk about what the person *can* do. This is a useful technique to try to avert potentially difficult situations.

Adding clues

We can help many people to understand their environment more fully, if we use additional clues to clarify our messages:

1. Use natural gestures more, such as pointing, appropriate facial expression.
2. Use a formal sign system such as the Makaton Vocabulary.
3. Pictures can be used to indicate to someone what the message is about, where they are going, what they are going to do, who is coming to see them, and so on. These can begin as single pictures,

and be developed into picture boards or books.
4. A formal symbol system (eg Makaton or Bliss) can be used in the same way.
5. Some people have difficulty understanding pictures, so objects can be selected to represent activities, people and events. These can be shown to the person to indicate what they are about to do. If the person has sensory impairments, objects are doubly valuable as they can use their sense of touch to explore the object and gain information from it. Thus a swimming costume could be given to someone to show them they are about to go swimming.

Whenever objects, pictures or symbols are being used, it is important to plan ahead. Think about which messages and topics you are likely to be communicating about, and gather the objects and pictures in advance.

You can also make a collection of objects and pictures. These can be for general use, or you could have a box with an individual's name on it, containing pictures or objects representing things about which they may want to communicate.

Using objects and pictures to help someone understand our messages is also a useful step to developing expressive skills. The person with learning disabilities can use the same items to begin to send clearer messages to us about what they would like to do, and thus begin to make choices.

Expressive skills

There are two main types of message that people can send: those which are intentional, and those which are unintentional.

Intentional messages are those where a person has an idea they want to express, decides how he/she would like to express it, and then tries to do so. They may try to speak, sign, or gesture.

Unintentional messages can be seen as a person's natural reaction to his environment, and his feelings. For example, someone may start crying because they are in pain, without intending to communicate that to anyone else. However we may work out that something is wrong, simply from the crying behaviour.

Many people with severe learning disabilities are at the stage of sending unintentional messages. They send very few intentional messages, because they have not learned a means of communication. Others have begun to send intentional messages, but they have developed their own code of signals, which we may find hard to understand.

Unconventional messages: recognise and value them

Just because the signals some people send may be unconventional, we must not discard them as unimportant. If we can learn to recognise them they can be a key to an individual's future development, acceptance, and participation.

We can keep a record, called a personal communication profile. Part of one might look like this:

PERSONAL COMMUNICATION PROFILE	
What is the message?	How is it expressed?
I need the toilet.	Rocks on chair.
I am hungry.	Chews and salivates.
I don't want this.	Pushes item away.
I am happy.	Smiles and rocks.

As in all aspects of working with people with learning disabilities, information should be sought from as many different people and settings as possible, as communication can vary greatly with different people and in different contexts.

Once a chart like this is made up, it can be circulated to people who are likely to need or want to communicate with the person. This improves the chances of them being able to have a successful, enjoyable interaction. It can be invaluable to new staff and people not seen every day, such as therapists, social club members, shopkeepers.

Sometimes a person will be sending a very clear message, but through challenging behaviour. This should be included in the list. Check Chapter 8 for ideas on handling this situation.

Developing new skills

I have already stressed the need for people to see communication as useful and enjoyable if they are to have the motivation to communicate.

Other major considerations are:

What will they communicate about?
Choose vocabulary which is seen by the person to be interesting and worthwhile.

Choose vocabulary which, if the person does attempt to communicate it, can often be responded to. Swimming or horse riding are thus not good choices for first vocabularies, because most of the time we would have to respond to the person's request by saying no. This will not encourage them to see communication as enjoyable and useful, whereas asking for a drink, or to go upstairs, could always be responded to.

How will they communicate it?
The main considerations are:
• As many people as possible need to be able to understand the person's attempts at communication, to prevent frustration and disillusion developing.
• People with limited communication skills are initially likely to be more motivated to use a simple form of communication, such as pointing to an

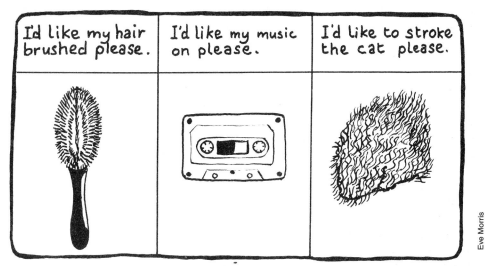

I'd like my hair brushed please.	I'd like my music on please.	I'd like to stroke the cat please.

Eve Morris

An example of an object board: the hairbrush, tape cassette and piece of fur are glued on.

object or picture. A more complex system, such as speech or signs, can be introduced when the person has learned that the communication process is worthwhile, and is motivated to develop this.

Objects, pictures and symbols

For these reasons objects, picture or symbol charts and books are proving very successful. An "object board" is shown in the illustration above.

These forms of communication have the advantage that they can be easily recognised by most people wherever the person goes.

The main consideration for these forms of communication is that the chart, board or book needs to be available to the person at all times. Duplicates can be left in frequently visited settings, and everyone who comes into contact with the person should be told of their existence, and how they will be used.

Sign systems

Sign systems have been used extensively with people with learning disabilities. The most widely used, and most useful, is the Makaton vocabulary. However, it should be remembered that for a sign system to be successful, the following factors are essential:

1. People in all settings that the person visits need to be familiar with the vocabulary, and be kept up to date with the signs each person knows.

2. If someone's fine motor control prevents them from producing exact signs, everyone needs to be informed of the variations and respond to their best efforts.

3. Families and care staff need to use the signs themselves, regularly and consistently.

If these considerations can be met, sign systems can be very valuable. If they are not met, people who have been taught signs often fail to use them spontaneously, or become even more frustrated when their attempts at communication are not recognised.

Clearer speech

The oral movements we make when

speaking are the fastest and most precise movements any part of our body ever makes. For this reason, there are many factors which can impede someone's ability to produce clear speech. Teaching a person to improve the clarity of their speech is a highly complex task, and depending upon the reasons for the difficulty, it may be a very long slow process.

Some people with learning disabilities make attempts at speech, or even speak in sentences, but these can be unclear, particularly to strangers. In this situation, we should always encourage the speech, but it is often of great benefit to the person if we offer them a supplementary means of communication. This can be objects, pictures, symbols or signs, to be used when a listener cannot understand the spoken message. Again, this increases the chance that a person will experience successful interactions, and reduces the sensation of pressure they may feel, sometimes preventing a build-up of frustration which can result in episodes of challenging behaviour.

Repetitive speech (echolalia) deserves particular mention. Some people with learning disabilities speak mainly in words or phrases which they use again and again. Sometimes it can appear that the phrases are being used appropriately, other times at random.

It is important for us to realise that we may be misled by either the quantity or the clarity of the person's speech into having expectations which are much too high. People with this type of speech often have very limited ability to understand what is said to them. They have learned the phrases simply as strings of sounds, not as meaningful words, and therefore cannot use the words outside the phrase,

nor with real meaning. We must be aware of this, and inform other people who interact with the person.

> There is no point in working to improve an individual's communication skills if we do not recognise that we will probably need to create opportunities for him to use the skills – and make sure we can respond.

Points to remember

1. Make sure the person has a way of attracting our attention to let us know he has something to say. Some people do not realise they need to attract our attention, and just sit in their chair signing or speaking. When no one responds, they may either become frustrated, or decide that communication is a waste of time and give up.

2. Have supplementary communication equipment such as objects and pictures available at all times.

3. Adjust what you say and do, to make it clearer, and be aware of how easy it is for people with learning disabilities to misunderstand what is said to them.

4. Use additional clues to make sure people understand what we are saying.

5. Be aware of the consequences when people misunderstand.

6. Be on the look-out for opportunities for people to have enjoyable, successful interactions, and *create* them if necessary.

7. Improve communication between the different settings which the person visits, like the day centre and the hostel. This will increase our knowledge of an individual, and should result in more ideas for topics of conversation and a clearer idea of their level of communication and understanding.

CHAPTER 6
Sight and hearing problems

Anne Clarke Kehoe

• The importance of full professional assessment • The effects of sensory impairment • Common causes of sight or hearing problems • Signs to look out for • How to help people with communication • Hearing aids and spectacles

Large numbers of people with learning disabilities have added problems with communicating their wants, needs and feelings, because they have impaired sight or hearing.

The general term *sensory impairment* describes the situation where any of the five senses - vision, hearing, smell, touch, and taste are not functioning to their potential. We use our senses primarily to gather information about the world around us. From this we learn about our environment, ourself and other people. We store the sensory information and use the memory to help us recognise sensations we have experienced before.

The two main sensory handicaps are hearing and visual impairment. Various studies have shown that up to 45% of people with severe and profound learning disabilities may have sensory impairments of some kind.

However, in many services for this client group, obtaining thorough assessment is difficult, particularly if the people involved are unable to cooperate with conventional forms of assessment.

This can often mean we expect too much of people. No allowances are made for sensory impairments until they are formally diagnosed.

Do 45% of the people in your service have recognised sensory impairments? Probably not, which may mean that many have sensory difficulties you are unaware of, and are not making allowances for.

Assessment

Despite the difficulties which can sometimes be encountered when trying to obtain assessment for people with learning disabilities, we must be persistent. Every person has the right to specialist services.

Most services for people living in the community can be obtained through the GP. Children and young adults should receive assessments through the education service. If the person is in the care of a consultant, they should be able to make a referral.

It should be noted that services vary from area to area, so not all the following services may be available in all areas.

Services available for visual assessment

Clinical Assessment aims to examine the structure of the eye, how well it reacts to different stimuli, whether there are any medical conditions affecting the eye, and the consequences for the person's vision.

This can be done by a local optician, or ophthalmology or optometry service at a hospital.

Functional Assessment aims to discover how well a person can utilise the vision they have. It would give information about the size and shape of a person's visual field, their best visual distance, optimum positioning, colour contrast problems, and so on. This can be done by:

Specialist in a low vision clinic
Social services technical officer
Specialist social worker
Peripatetic teaching specialist from local education authority.

The two assessments complement one another, so both should be sought.

Services for hearing assessment

Hearing or audiological assessment aims to identify the degree of hearing loss, ie: the level of sound a person can and cannot hear; and the type of hearing loss – what sort of sounds the person can hear (eg high or low pitch sounds).

These assessments are usually carried out by the local audiology service. This may lead to a referral to the Ear, Nose and Throat (ENT) department at a hospital.

The assessments used vary in the amount of cooperation that is required from the individual. There are specialist assessments which can be done under anaesthetic, but these are obviously not done frequently, and are only available at certain locations in the UK.

What are the effects of sensory impairment?

• A reduction in information received
• Problems of understanding activities, objects and words.
• A limited, distorted or inaccurate perception of the environment.

Many of us have experienced the sensation of not being able to hear clearly what is being said, perhaps at a noisy party. We may also have been blindfolded, or in a totally dark place. As a rule, we cope very badly with this. Most people find these experiences distressing.

Sensory impairments can cause:

• Isolation
• Difficulty making relationships
• Lack of social skills
• Mobility problems
• Diminished ability to learn
• Lack of awareness of your environment
• Lack of self awareness and self esteem
• Lack of confidence
• Withdrawal
• Lessened opportunity to participate in activities, and in the community
• Problems understanding other people's communication or feelings
• Other people seeing you as stupid or uncooperative.

There is also a higher incidence of self stimulatory, self injurious and ritualistic behaviours in people who have both sensory impairments and learning disabilities. As people with sensory handicaps attempt to adjust to their world as they perceive it, their behaviour may seem to us to be inappropriate, bizarre or even "challenging".

For example, a person with visual impairment may find that the only way they can get any visual stimulation is by poking their eyes quite hard.

The above factors are true for anyone with sensory impairments. However there are two important points to consider:

1. The problems faced by an individual increase according to how severe the impairment is, and how many senses are involved. People with severe learning disabilities are more likely to have more

than one sense involved, than people without learning disabilities.

2. People who have sensory impairments, who do not have learning difficulties, attempt to cope with their disability by using their other senses more fully, and learning new, adapted skills. For people with learning disabilities, we know that learning new skills is, in itself, a problem. So we should never underestimate the effects of a combination of handicaps on the individual concerned.

Sight problems

Common physical causes of sight problems:
Malformation of the eye, the optic nerve or visual cortex in the brain
Glaucoma
Cataracts
Detached retina
Short/long sightedness.
Tunnel vision/peripheral vision
Squint
Eye drops; medication
Injury, including self injury
Epilepsy.

Common environmental causes of poor sight:
Lost/broken/dirty/unsuitable glasses
Seating position which doesn't make best use of vision
Lighting – too bright, too dim
Light reflected off surfaces
Lack of contrast, eg between object and table top
Items in front of eyes – hands, hair, mobiles...
Smoke, chlorine, hair spray.

Signs which MAY indicate a visual impairment:
The eye itself may be inflamed, or water.
It may be swollen,
move very rapidly,
or have frequent infections.

The person may
– be reluctant to open their eyes
– rub eyes, rock, blink rapidly, avoid light
– be clumsy, shuffle feet when walking
– be reluctant to move
– startle when approached
– be reluctant to move in strange places
– not bother to look for things
– explore things through touch
– fail to notice people or appear to take no notice of them, until they are very close
– become bored, anxious or irritable during tasks which are mainly visual.

Hearing problems

Common physical causes of hearing loss:
Malformation of the ear – narrow ear canal, immobile bones within ear, malfunction of auditory nervous system and/or auditory cortex in the brain
Perforated eardrum
Injury to ear including self injury
Wax in ears
Repeated ear infections
Medication
Tinnitus (ringing in the ears).

Common environmental causes of poor hearing:
Noise
Unsuitable/lost/ broken hearing aid
Batteries flat or tubes in aid blocked
Hat over ears
Headphones over ears
Fingers in ears/hands over ears.
Objects in ears, eg beads
Water in ears.

Signs which MAY indicate a hearing impairment:
The ear itself may be small, or have a narrow ear canal.
It may secrete excessive wax,
smell,
or have recurring infections.
The person may:
– pull, rub or poke his ears

– rock
– tilt head to listen
– startle when approached
– stare at sound source
– shout
– bang
– make very loud noises, or speak loudly
– have very distorted speech
– touch vibrating objects, eg speakers, washing machines
– fail to respond when spoken to (not necessarily all the time, as hearing may be directional if only one ear is affected, and/or some voices – eg women's voices – may be harder to decipher than men's lower voices)
– DISLIKE loud sounds (this may seem strange, but they can sound very distorted to someone with a hearing loss)
– fail to respond to certain people, voices, types of request.

We need to be aware that any of these signs MAY indicate a sensory difficulty. Hearing impairments may vary from day to day – often we assume that people are being a nuisance by deliberately not hearing when their hearing may be unreliable or they may usually be guessing at our meaning from other clues.

Notice that many of the items in the lists of causes are avoidable: hats, wax, seating position, reflected light, noise, and so on. These things should always be checked out first. Glasses should be cleaned every day, or they add to the problem rather than solve it!

We must also be wary of case notes which state "hearing and vision normal". If there is no evidence to support this – such as the result of a recent hearing test – we should not assume that it is necessarily correct, and should try to get a full assessment made. It is very hard to tell whether someone is able to make full use of their hearing and vision, especially if their mobility and communication are impaired. Many of the pointers which might indicate a sensory impairment would be missing for these people. For example we would not notice whether someone shuffled his feet, or held out his hands in front of him to check for obstacles, if he was not mobile.

Hearing aids

There are two main types of hearing aid currently available:

The body worn aid is used by a few people with very severe hearing loss.

The smaller "behind the ear" aid, available with different power levels, is the most widely used.

It is **essential** to remember that a hearing aid will not instantly solve all the problems a hearing impaired person has had. It will amplify every sound, not just speech, and many people find a hearing aid very distressing and confusing, not just for the first few days, but often for many months.

We must therefore consider how we introduce the aid to the person, and ensure we are familiar with how the aid works, and its maintenance.

1. The microphone. This must not be blocked by fingers, food, etc.

2. Switch.   O – Off
T – Transduction loop
M – Microphone (On)

The transduction loop switch can be used wherever this symbol is used, usually in theatres, churches, ticket offices, telephone kiosks. This will allow the person to hear the sound by radio link, much more clearly. Remember to return the switch to the M position afterwards, or if you wish to speak to the person!

3. Battery compartment.
Batteries last between 1 to 3 months

depending upon their type, and the amount of use. They should be kept, and returned to the issuing audiology department where they can be exchanged for new ones free of charge.

If the aid whistles when switched on, and with the volume turned up, the battery is charged. If you cannot get a whistle, it is dead.

4. Volume

To find the best volume setting, adjust the volume to the point just below where a whistle is heard. Check the whistle does not return if the person shakes his head. Observe the person to see if they seem comfortable with this volume.

5. Plastic tube

The sound passes through this tube, so it must be kept clean and flexible. It should be renewed regularly at the audiology clinic.

6. Ear mould

This is made for the individual, and cannot be worn by anyone else. The small

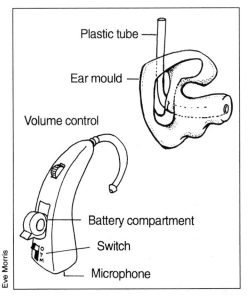

Plastic tube —

Ear mould —

Volume control

Battery compartment

Switch

Microphone

Eve Morris

"Behind the ear" hearing aid and ear mould.

hole at the end is where the sound enters the ear. If this becomes blocked with wax, the aid is much less efficient.

It is therefore essential that the person's ears are checked for wax by the GP every six months. Care staff should check and remove any wax obvious in the outer ear every day.

Introducing a new hearing aid

1. Try to prepare the person by getting them used to having something in or around their ears – sunglasses, headphones, cotton wool, even earrings!
2. When the aid arrives, allow the person to wear it for a few minutes, switched OFF. Then in a very quiet room, switch the aid on. **Make sure it does not whistle by pre-setting the volume in your own ear first.** Talk to the person for a few minutes, then remove the aid.

Very gradually build up the person's tolerance by allowing them to wear the aid a little longer each day, and increasing the situations in which they wear it.

A possible schedule is shown below.

Day 1: 3 mins; quiet room, aid switched off.
Day 2: 3 minutes; quiet room, aid on.
Day 3: 5 minutes; quiet room, aid on.
Days 4-8: Up to 30 mins; quiet room, aid on.
Day 9: 15 minutes; room with some background noise.
Days 10-20: Up to 1 hour; either setting.
Day 21: 2 x 1 hour; either setting.
Day 22: 2 x 1 hour;either setting.
Then add a short trip outdoors.

Continue to build up the programme very gradually. This will make it much more likely that someone will learn to accept the aid, and use it. Do not worry if you need to backtrack the programme for a while.

Finally, with both hearing aids and glasses, remember that one of the reasons they are rejected is simply that they hurt!

Check to see if there is a red area behind the ear: if so Vaseline and a small cotton wool pad may help. If necessary, leave the aid or glasses off for a few days.

Glasses can also cause soreness on the bridge of the nose. If the soreness persists, return to the optician and ask for them to be adjusted.

Points to remember

1. People with learning disabilities and sensory handicaps need to have great trust and confidence in their carers.

2. They will need very clear messages, possibly using objects or other props which allow them to make use of other senses. For example, if you want someone to choose whether they want to listen to a tape or do a jigsaw, hand them a cassette box and a piece of the puzzle so they can use their hands to add to your spoken words and make up for poor vision.

3. They will need more time to take in information, and to attempt to respond.

4. Great efforts must be made to create a very consistent environment. This includes keeping furniture and equipment in the same place, using the same simple words or objects to communicate and offer choices, and sticking to routines so that the person with learning disabilities knows what is happening and when.

5. We must try to be aware of the way the person may interpret his environment. This should include recognising that some bizarre or inappropriate behaviours may just be that person's best attempt to adapt to their distorted picture of the world.

6. Try to get full assessment for everyone.

7. There are probably many people with learning disabilities with undetected sensory impairments. We may need to start adjusting our expectations for them, and be more alert to visual and hearing difficulties.

8. Some causes of sensory impairments are avoidable; we should be alert to this.

9. Glasses and hearing aids are not always the answer, but if prescribed should be introduced carefully and maintained appropriately.

10. A person with hearing impairment will probably try to make better use of their visual skills and *vice versa*. So we need to make sure that both hearing and visual environments are as near ideal as we can possibly make them.

Resources

The following organisations produce excellent literature and offer training courses:

The Derbyshire Language Scheme. Mark Masidlover, Educational Psychology Service, Amber Valley & Erewash Area Education Office, Grosvenor Road, Ripley, Derby DE5 3JE.

Makaton Vocabulary Development Project. Mrs M Walker, Director, 31 Firwood Drive, Camberley, Surrey.

SENSE (National Deaf/Blind and Rubella Association), 11-13 Clifton Terrace, London N4. Tel: 071 278 1005.

Royal National Institute for the Blind, 224 Great Portland St, London W1N 6AA. Tel: 071 388 1266.

Royal National Institute for the Deaf, 105 Gower St, London WC1E 6AH. Tel: 071 387 8033.

Further reading

Making sense of the world. A guide for Carers. Helen Bradley and Bob Snow. Published by SENSE (address above).

Understanding and responding to difficult behaviour and *Developing communication skills.* Video assisted training packages in the Bringing People Back Home series, available from Outset Publishing, Unit 8 Conqueror Industrial Estate, Moorhurst Road, St Leonards-on-Sea, East Sussex TN38 9NA. Tel: 0424 854124.

CHAPTER 7

Challenging behaviour

Sheila Barrett

• What do we mean by challenging behaviour? • Gathering information from past and present about the person and their environment • Describing exactly what happens, in what circumstances, can help us to understand why • A helpful response – planning and following it through consistently

The term "challenging behaviour" is used so often that most care staff would say that almost everyone they work with has some form of "challenging" behaviour. In fact, we are sometimes so quick to label people, that those who try to express dissatisfaction or communicate a need through means which we would see as different or abnormal, find themselves labelled as "difficult" or "challenging". Once this has happened they can acquire a permanent label, and what inevitably follows is that they are seen as people who are difficult, rather than victims of a service which is unable to understand or respond successfully to their needs.

What is challenging?

"Challenging behaviour" can mean different things to different people at different times. To some extent, what gets defined as challenging can depend on the care staff's own level of toleration, which may or may not be affected by their values and prejudices, together with the stresses they are experiencing at that particular time. Some staff, for reasons such as:

• dedicated caring feelings
• poor supervision
• fear of being without a job
• lack of training and support,

put up with situations that are very abusive both to themselves and people with learning disabilities, and consider it to be a normal part of their work. But faced with these situations, staff can quickly be forced into a position where they blame the person and see them as the problem, instead of recognising the impossible situation in which they have been put, or seeing that the service is at fault for failing to provide the insight or resources needed.

One professional's definition of challenging behaviour is that "which services find extremely difficult to manage".[1] The author estimates that between 10 and 15 out of 100,000 people with a learning disability show such behaviour, which includes physical aggression toward others and/or the environment, and self injury.

A further definition is "behaviour of such intensity, frequency or duration that the physical safety of the person or others is likely to be placed in serious jeopardy, or behaviour which is likely to seriously limit or delay access to and use of ordinary community facilities"[2].

For those working in direct contact with people with a learning disability, what is important is the strength of the behaviour itself and the impact it has on others.

There is an interaction between the environment and the behaviour itself, so that at times one influences the other to such an extent that the behaviour is seen as challenging. For example, there may be times when any sort of disagreement or refusal to do what is asked or expected may be considered challenging. This could well happen in situations where too few staff are expected to achieve too much. At other times, the behaviour may be very serious, but staff will not register it as challenging enough to recognise that they need help. This could be because morale is low, or because they have found helpful ways of handling the situation.

There is no doubt about the seriousness of many challenging behaviours and the human response they evoke. To see someone gradually biting away their lip, gouging their eye, or engaging in aggression which leaves others injured and scarred, leads staff to immediately run or try to restrain. Facing this type of situation on a daily basis can be draining on staff if they are not well supervised, and trained, to respond in ways that are supportive to both the person and to themselves.

Where this type of support is lacking, care staff are often told to "use their common sense", an approach which obviously has not worked in the past . This approach is also likely to add to care staff's sense of failure and further diminish their sense of worth and skill.

Towards understanding

When we are trying to understand difficult behaviour we need to assess the whole situation, not just the behaviour or the environment but how they interact. It is also important to piece together a picture of the social and physical environments where people have lived in the past, including the "politics" or philosophy of care at that time, and where possible detail about the individual's past physical and mental health.

Information from the present will help us to understand the current factors that are influencing the person's behaviour. Such factors include **social factors** such as:
• the types of behaviours which are acceptable - the rules for living, and the examples the person has around from other people;
• how well the person is understood, and the level of skill and understanding of those around them;
• the quality of their interaction with other people;
• who the significant people are in that person's life.

Information about **physical surroundings** will help us to understand:
• how people spend their time;
• how much opportunity they have for meaningful activity in stimulating surroundings;
• how often they have pleasurable and interesting activities or experiences.

Information from the past is important in helping us understand:
• the person's learning experiences, how they communicate and get their needs met;
• the major events which have influenced their lives, and attempts at treatment that have worked or not worked;
• anything we can learn about times when the person was reported as being reasonably content.

Political factors include:
• What were the predominant service models at that time, and

• how did they reflect the attitudes and behaviour of the society towards the person? Especially,

• how might being a woman, being black or from an ethnic minority, being homosexual, affect how others treated them?

Information on the individual's **physical and mental health** should include:

• Has the person had any serious medical conditions? Do they cause pain, irritation , discomfort?

• Are they taking or have they in the past taken any medication on a regular basis?

• What sort of diagnoses have been made in the past? Have any treatments or interventions worked or not worked?

Why and when

Bringing all this information together will help us to look at three areas which are important when we are trying to understand difficult behaviour and what it means to that person. From such an assessment we can tease out:

1. The function that a behaviour serves for that person. The question we are asking ourselves is: "What is the relationship between the behaviour and what happens as a result of the behaviour? In other words, what does the person achieve from behaving in this way?

For example, by hitting their head, someone may get much wanted and needed social or physical contact from a staff member, or they might get left alone and appreciate the time alone.

2. Indicators in the environment which signal to the person that the behaviour is likely to be successful in meeting their need. In this instance we are interested in what was happening before the behaviour occurred. In the example above, it may be that the staff member being within the person's field of vision is an indication to

that person that if they hit their head then they are likely to receive contact, so it acts as a kind of trigger.

3. General factors in the environment which increase stress for that person, may make it more likely that the difficult behaviour will occur. Examples might be noise levels, heat, crowding – we all know what it is like to be hot and irritable.

Looking at these three areas can help us understand both why the behaviour is occurring and what it means to that person, and also under what conditions it is more likely to occur. Information that is pooled together and used in this way will help us distinguish between challenging behaviour and the day-to-day obstinacy and irritability which is everyone's right. From our powerful position, we need to be aware that at times we try to make people with learning disabilities into super-human or non-human beings who behave placidly, are obedient and sexless.

This is not true of us, of course. Some days we are happy and calm. Equally there are times when we are so fed up with our persistence at a task that we throw the lot down or kick it into the air. People with learning disabilities share these same experiences, which may be exacerbated by poor communication (their own, or sometimes that of the staff).

This is not to deny that there are instances in people's lives which warrant extra understanding and help on our part. To appreciate this, we need to consider the learning histories and capabilities of many people with severe learning difficulties, as well as those of care services.

Finding out why

Why do people behave in ways that are challenging?

A commonly held notion about difficult behaviour, whatever sort, is that it is "attention seeking". This belief may originate from our experiences with children, but research shows that in the adult world people behave in ways that we find difficult, not always to gain attention from others, but for a number of reasons, each of which is very personal to that individual. Researchers and practitioners alike are now putting forward the idea that difficult behaviour is a means of communicating various needs, and therefore has a number of different "functions". The most common have been identified as follows:

1. To AVOID demands or escape difficult situations. Examples are numerous and commonplace. For instance:
• A task presented to the person may be too complex; it may be beyond the person's capabilities, they don't possess the skills to carry it out.
• The person may not understand the language used, or the instructions may be vague, unclear, too complicated, or in too many steps given all at once.
• It may be that the person has an extreme dislike of an activity, or worse still a great fear of a situation or person, perhaps because of a bad experience in the past.

2. To GAIN access to interesting things to do. People are often bored and desperate for activity (other chapters in this book give plenty of ideas for participation in daily living, and activities). If someone's behaviour results in them being drawn into an activity, it may become their way of making things happen around them.

3. Sensory stimulation
In the absence of things to do, people may create their own stimulation, through what are often called "stereotyped behaviours". Typically these are behaviours which are continually repeated, such as spinning, hand-flapping and rocking. One theory is that some self-

injuring behaviours are continued because they release hormones into the bloodstream which reduce pain and discomfort.

4. To gain attention
Many people with a learning disability have little contact with others. They may have few and small family networks; staff contact may be poor and there may be much competition for what little there is. Because the levels of interaction are often well below normal, people may use difficult behaviour to secure some sort of contact, be it positive or negative.

What we have to remember about these broad categories is that they give us an indication as to why someone is behaving in a particular way, but there is a lot of other information, as indicated above, which needs to be accumulated in order to determine what the behaviour means for that particular person. The same behaviour may serve different functions for different individuals, depending on their needs, their circumstances and the response they get.

Many care staff find it difficult to accept that some of the aggression staff experience from service users may be unintentional, not "done on purpose", but this *is* so. If we really wanted to hurt someone else, most of us have learned that there are places in the body to hit where it really hurts. People with learning disabilities typically lash out indiscriminately.

Our response

The first place to start when responding to difficult behaviour, is for staff to acknowledge the position of power from which they and their services operate, and the potential they have for abusing that power. This is not helped by some of the unwritten rules which exist in many care services. For instance, there may be pressure "not to rock the boat" which

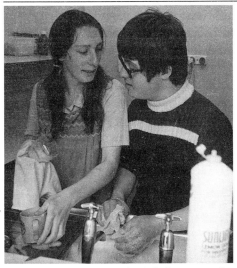

Photo: Mencap

People are often bored and desperate for activity: challenging behaviour may be their way of making things happen around them.

means that staff are put in a position where they are controllers of what are seen to be difficult people.

Because of these factors, and others such as communication, it is important to be aware of the methods we use when we respond and intervene in difficult situations. Of course there are times when we need someone to do as we say, for example for their own safety, but if someone is screaming with pain, thirst or frustration at a task which is too difficult, how can we justify a response that punishes or ignores that person's needs?

The next step is to define the behaviour, and begin to measure it. Defining and measuring it clearly will help us to:

• intervene at consistent points;
• see whether our interventions work; and
• monitor changes in the behaviour.

Having defined some of the reasons why people behave as they do, we must not then be comforted into thinking that the remedy is easy. This is not always the case because someone may have used this method of communication for many

years, and to break the pattern is extremely difficult.

We also need to attend to other quality areas in the person's life; wiping out the behaviour which we see as difficult is not enough. We must ensure that the person is given *appropriate* means by which they can communicate and have their needs understood, and they need to live in interesting environments which meet their needs for stimulation.

The role of care staff

1. The accurate collection of information.
Care staff have more day-to-day contact than other professionals, and are therefore in a position to know the person best. Collecting information accurately is vitally important if we are to gain an honest and true account of what is going on in that person's life. It will also lead to consistency in applying any procedures, and so increase the likelihood that interventions will actually work.

2. Using information positively
Information needs to be used in a non-punitive manner, so that everyone gets a clear picture of what is happening and all the different factors at work. If inform-ation is used by managers of care staff to blame them for the difficult behaviour of the people they work with, then this will eventually defeat the trust and effective-ness of the staff team. We all need to use information in a healthy way which enables us to get a clear and accurate account of what is going on. If things are going well, there is reason to celebrate; if not, staff should still congratulate themselves on being honest, and look for ways of thinking through the problem.

3. Following procedures of intervention
Where procedures have been designed, in order to try and change someone's

behaviour, they must be followed carefully and consistently by care staff. Many procedures are designed to give consistent messages to people or teach them specific ways of doing something. It is care staff who are in the position to ensure that this happens. So often it is said that "nothing seems to work" when in fact it may be that staff are responding inconsistently or sometimes not at all. It is vital to agree to one procedure and then follow it exactly.

4. Openly and honestly acknowledging your part in responding to difficult behaviour

Care staff need to describe an honest and accurate picture of what is happening in the service – to "say how it is". So, for example, if staffing levels are low and there really was not time to fill in the information that was required from your shift, then you must say so. Information remembered two days later will be inaccurate and will not be helpful to anyone in the long term. A necessary condition for this honesty is that managers treat information positively without blaming anyone, as described above.

5. Offering positive role models

To people with a learning disability, care staff provide role models for both positive (appropriate, socially acceptable) and negative (unacceptable) behaviours. For example, if female staff are harassed by male staff while on duty then it is likely that this will be seen as a model of interaction between men and women. When a man then uses harassment as a means of relating to female members of staff or the public, their behaviour will be seen as challenging.

6. Accentuate the positive. Encouraging and teaching socially appropriate behaviours will increase the likelihood of the individual being understood.

An important role of care staff is to encourage and adhere to programmes which develop people's skills and chances of being understood and accepted by others. Staff will need to use a combination of modelling these behaviours and carefully following the programme designed for the individual.

Points to remember

1. Difficult behaviour is difficult partly because people with learning disabilities have had to live in difficult environments, where they have been ignored, bored or misunderstood.
2. People with severe learning difficulties or communication problems have often not been able to ask effectively for what they want.
3. It is most unlikely that challenging behaviour is directed at you personally, or that it is the person's fault, even if it seems that way.
4. Trying to figure out what purpose it serves for the individual could put you, as a staff team, on the road to finding alternative, acceptable ways for the person to be in control of what happens to them.

References

1. Kiernan (1987) *Dilemmas: services for mentally handicapped people with challenging behaviours.* Paper at BIMH Conference, Llantrisant, Wales.
2. Emerson, Barrett, Bell, Cummings, McCool, Toogood, Mansell (1987) *Developing services for people with severe learning difficulties and challenging behaviours.* University of Kent at Canterbury, Institute of Social and Applied Psychology.

Resources

Understanding and responding to difficult behaviour and *Developing communication skills.* Video assisted training packages in the Bringing People Back Home series, available from Outset Publishing, Unit 8 Conqueror Industrial Estate, Moorhurst Road, St Leonards-on-Sea, East Sussex TN38 9NA. Tel: 0424 854124.

CHAPTER 8

Sharing the tasks of daily living

Sheila Barrett and Zenia Wainwright-Melnyk

• Do things with, not for people • Provide opportunities and encourage people to join in • Break tasks down into stages • Assess the help each individual needs • How to organise your time and theirs • Useful charts

Why do we want people with learning disabilities to join in with the everyday tasks and activities of ordinary life? And why do we need to work at making opportunities for them to do so?

In the past, services for people with learning disabilities have discouraged them from sharing the jobs that are generated through their day to day living. All catering and laundry was done centrally, and domestic staff were brought in to carry out cleaning and tidying-up activities. People experienced things happening to them and around them with little knowledge or control over those things. For example, they may have had

• to get up at a set time in the morning when they perhaps felt like a lie in;

• tea given to them when they were not thirsty, and no drink available when they needed one;

• a three course meal presented when all they wanted was a snack.

In other words, services and staff decided what was best for them and helped them accordingly. This type of service, although well intentioned and

motivated with the aims of protection, care and concern, often assumed that people with learning disabilities could not contribute to the running of their lives. However, research and experience have now shown us that people with learning disabilities have and can learn skills which can enable them to make decisions and be involved in their own daily life.

The new community based settings for people with learning disabilities largely reflect this knowledge, and care staff are expected to involve people in daily household activities.

Many job descriptions state such expectations, and most staff are enthusiastic about this new emphasis, but all too often services let staff down by failing to give them the training, structures and information they need in order to get the process going. Our experience is that involving people in these activities does not just happen, it is a product of much planning and support.

What is participation?

Just what do we mean by involvement and participation, and how is it different from other activities like teaching?

61

Participation is:

• Staff doing things *with* people.

• People with learning disabilities taking a positive part in all the activities of day to day living.

   Sharing everyday tasks which are appropriate to the person's lifestyle does not necessarily mean a fifty-fifty split in carrying out the activity, but rather that the task gets done with the staff member giving whatever assistance is necessary for it to happen. At times the contribution of the care staff may be 95 per cent, at others it may only be two per cent, but at all times the staff member will be attending to the task 100 per cent of the time, either through watching or doing the activity.

Participation is not:

• Staff doing things *for* people.

• Teaching a new skill. In the past, some staff have confused participation with teaching, but in teaching the aim is for the person to become independent in a skill, whereas the aim of participation is that the person is involved in the activity. As a result of participating the person may or may not learn.

• Training people to be independent. It is important to be clear about this because severely disabled people can be helped to participate when they might never be able to do things on their own.

Why is it important?

It is through active participation that we experience variety in life, and without variety we cannot begin to make real and informed choices about our lives. Taking part also increases our chances of inter-acting with others in more meaningful and purposeful ways and on a more equal footing; rather than being the person that is "spoken at" or "done to". This increases the possibility of gaining respect from others around us, perhaps being seen as someone who is capable and entitled to exert some control over what goes on around us. Being seen by others as someone who is taking part increases our value among those people and promotes opportunities to attract others into our lives. Altogether, participation increases our quality of life.

The role of care staff

• Participation depends on the number of opportunities care staff create. Therefore it is the responsibility of services to generate a wide range of activities, and to organise and create ways of working which always include the client.

• Participation needs two way interaction because the person is unable to participate until you give them the chance. You will need to do your share of the task as well as oversee their contribution.

• Judging the level of help given is a staff responsibility. It is the role of the care staff to gauge the level of assistance, giving neither too much nor too little help. It relies on staff sensitivity to those they care for and to the surroundings. It can be viewed as a problem-solving activity which invites care staff to find ways of attracting and maintaining the person's interest.

Obstacles

It is all too easy for unsupported staff to have their best efforts destroyed by what they see as failure. The following situations are common:

1. People refuse to join in activities and we don't know what to do.
• First of all we need to check: Can the person understand the instructions given? If not we must change them so that they

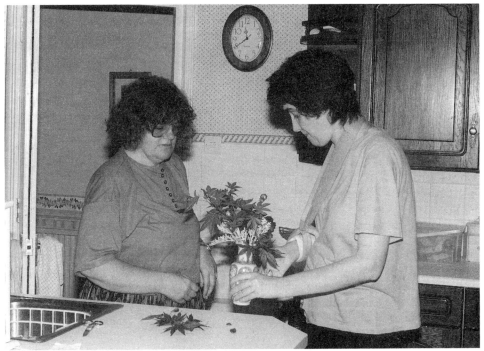

Photo: Sue Benson

Participation is staff doing things with people, sharing everyday tasks.

do (see Chapter 5). For instance, if you have given a verbal instruction and there does not appear to be any response, try miming or pointing to what needs to be done. Give any other type of clue or prompt you can think of that would be of help to the person understanding what you expect of them.

• Are they physically capable, for example of grasping the saucepan or turning the cooker dial?

• Have we made the activity enjoyable, inviting and fun? A sense of humour is a great help; reprimands and harsh instructions will put people off.

• Where people show little initiative in asking to join in an activity or indeed resist it, we need to ask ourselves:

Do they really want to watch the world go by, around and past them? Or have they learned through failure (for example if past instructions were too difficult), or through constantly having things done for them, that participation is fruitless? In this case, finding things we know the person can succeed at will be vital.

2. We give so much help in carrying out the task that we feel we might as well do it ourselves, and wonder what is the use of such an exercise.

At these times we need to bear in mind that even when the level of assistance given by staff is great, we still have to create opportunities to engage the person's attention, for example through smelling the aroma of food cooking, feeling the texture of a dough, pulling the plug out of the sink and hearing and seeing the water bubbling away, adding the bubble bath and watching the bubbles form, turning the oven alarm off when the cooking is finished.

3. We ask ourselves: What difference does it make anyway? Nobody really knows; do the managers really care? Do the people themselves really care?

Often we are given very little information about how well we are doing. Our managers may not recognise or acknowledge our achievements and efforts. To overcome this we need to keep our own tally of the number of opportunities we create in a day for a person, and the number that are taken up. In this way we can end our shift with a measure of achievement and a better idea of where we need to concentrate our efforts next time. An opportunity to share this information with other staff gives further recognition of our work and a chance to solve some of the difficulties we encounter.

4. We concentrate on getting the work done fast and we find ourselves saying "Surely it's quicker to do it myself".

How many times have you whispered this under your breath as you have struggled to involve someone in an activity? But does it really matter if it takes an hour to do the washing up, when the only alternative for the client is to sit in a chair and wait for the next meal?

5. We think people have too many disabilities to participate, and it might be kinder to do the activities for them.

This way of thinking leads us back into the old ways, which deprive people of any choice or control over their lives. There are always parts of an activity that a client can do, even if they cannot be involved in all of it.

Sometimes we find it difficult to see which steps in a task they can participate in, because we think of it as one continuous activity. For example we make cups of tea so often we overlook the fact that pouring milk into a cup does not involve any risk with a hot kettle. We need to break the task down so that at the very least they can do some bits and be encouraged to attend and watch other bits. You will never know what people are able to do unless you give them opportunities to try out new experiences.

6. We think our staffing levels are too low for us to give the levels of interaction that may be required.

This is often true, but there are always ways of planning our time so that rather than give up completely, we give some to individuals and some to group participation activities. Even ideal staff ratios never seem to be enough, and indeed research has shown that when we have too many staff on duty then we tend to talk to each other, rather than talk or interact with people with learning disabilities. Of course it is important to talk to other members of staff during the day, but sometimes this reflects how difficult or boring we find our attempts to communicate and understand the people we work with, so that the two way process of communication becomes one way from us to them (see Chapter 5).

7. We question the relevance of people doing a task when they do not appear to understand.

This dilemma is best illustrated with an example. Joe needs physical assistance to do the vacuuming and it would seem that he is unable to recognise when the vacuuming needs to be done. What is the benefit of him carrying out this task when he may not even know what dust or dirt is?

The issue here is: does he somehow have to learn the difference between clean and dirty in a "theoretical" way before he does the cleaning in his own home? Might it not be more beneficial for him to learn about differences "on the job". Could it be that he really enjoys the noise of the vacuum cleaner, or the backward and forward movement of the cleaning action and that this is enough to make it a worthwhile activity for him? Does he really have to be intellectually capable of understanding every activity?

8. Often care staff get caught in the dilemma of asking themselves "Should participation be a matter of choice? Or are there some tasks that are not negotiable."

A common proposition put forward is that if we had the choice, would we really choose to do the washing up and all the other domestic activities that are essential to living? Would we not rather sit back and have someone else do them for us?

We have to remind ourselves when questioning in this way that if we were in that position then we would probably have created lots of other, more stimulating activities in which to be involved. For someone with learning disabilities, is lying in bed until noon really a choice when there is no other activity on offer which they might find interesting or enjoyable? Is the "choice" of lying in bed or sitting in the lounge "waiting" all morning for lunch, really a choice at all?

How to help

Now we have defined what participation is and why it is an important part of any service, and also looked at the role of care staff in making it happen, it is time to focus on giving the right amount and type of help. There are six steps to be taken:

1. Identifying opportunities
2. Creating opportunities
3. Preparation
4. Breaking the activity down into stages
5, Assessing the client's skills in carrying out the activity, and determining the amount of help required
6. Carrying out the task, giving the amount of help identified.

Each of these steps will now be individually considered.

1. Identifying opportunities

Most of the activities that make up our day-to-day lives fall into two categories: things we have to do and don't necessarily enjoy (for most of us these are domestic chores) and things we enjoy (usually social and leisure activities). When we start to identify opportunities in a client's environment, we need to ensure that we have some of both categories.

One starting point may be to list the activities that we undertake in our own day-to-day living. Also, look around the environment where you work:

• Who picks up the post and opens envelopes?

• Who answers the telephone?

• Who uses the stereo? Who changes channels on the TV or radio?

• Who switches lights on and off?

• Who draws the curtains night and morning?

• Who waters the plants and takes the dead leaves off?

• Who gets cleaning materials out of the cupboard? Who puts them back?

• Who pulls the plug out after washing up?

• Who closes the microwave door, and switches it on and off?

• Can you find more opportunities to add to this list?

2. Creating opportunities

If you find it difficult to identify opportunities in the environment, then an alternative to just giving up is to look towards making life more interactive by creating them. For instance if there have been no phone calls during the day, can the person ring someone they want to talk to? Is there someone or some place they would really like to visit? Has the person had the experience of finding various channels on the radio and determining favourites?

Keeping Track

Name _____ Week ending _____

✓ = participation in activity
⊘ offered opportunity but refused

MEALS	M	T	W	T	F	S	S	Total
Cooked breakfast								
Cooked lunch								
Prepared snack								
Cooked evening meal								
Laid table								

WASHING UP	M	T	W	T	F	S	S	Total
Cleared table								
Washed up								
Used dishwasher								
Dried up								
Put dishes away								

SHOPPING	M	T	W	T	F	S	S	Total
Contributed to shopping list								
Did big shop in supermarket								
Bought fruit, veg, meat etc. from specialist shops								
Put shopping away								
Bought personal goods								

Part of the Keeping Track[1] form which can be used to keep records of participation in activities. Other sections include Gardening and Maintenance, Housework, Clothes, Trips out, Work, Day activities.

Could you go and try out different perfumes/aftershaves at a department store, for a future gift? Are there different kinds of hand cream they could try on their hands? If the person likes coffee, could you put together a "Good Coffee Guide" for your locality by visiting, sampling and rating all the coffee shops in the area? Are there areas in the person's individual plan that need expanding?

Another consideration may be to think of ways of adapting equipment to enable the person to participate: for example someone who has problems with coordination could use an electric toothbrush. Once you have identified or made opportunities the next step is to work out how you can make them accessible to each individual.

3. Preparation
Preparation refers to what the care worker needs to do to ensure that the scene is set for participation. Being prepared minimises the risk of confusion and chaos when you are involved in an activity. Here are a few examples. Can you think of others?

• In the winter months it can be very cold for a person sitting in a wheelchair. You may have developed a sweat in pushing the wheelchair but the client may be very cold indeed. Part of your preparation will need to take this into account by ensuring that they have warm clothing.

• You may want to limit the number of possible interruptions by ensuring that someone else is responsible for answering the phone or the door.

• It may be important that there are no others around, for example in the kitchen area when you are cooking. You may need to make other arrangements for other people.

• It may be that for someone who initially can only concentrate on an activity for a short period of time, you have to have everything ready. Perhaps at breakfast, for example, the cereals, milk, bread should be on the table ready for the person to start by serving themselves.

• You may want to plan a trip out for someone who uses a wheelchair. For this you will need to work out a route and a venue that is wheelchair accessible.

4. Breaking the activity down into stages
In order to assist a client confidently it is desirable to work out the stages in the task beforehand. To do this you will need an opportunity to go through the activity, making notes of the chunks into which it could be divided. Take for example, "Doing the washing". The stages are likely to be:

Stage of task	Skills needed
1. Sorting the pile of washing	
2. Loading the washing machine	
3. Pouring the washing powder	
4. Setting and starting the machine	
5. Unloading the machine	
6. Folding laundry ready for ironing	

You will need to be familiar with all the actions that are required in order to carry out the task, and to think about what sort of skills are required. For example, the ability to sort into colours; fine movements to select the right washing option on the machine; a steady hand to pour in the powder. You could write these in the boxes to help you remember.

5. Assessing the individual's skills and the amount of assistance required to carry out the task.
When assessing someone's skills to carry out an activity, start by asking whether they are physically capable of performing the various actions. All too often, it is assumed that people who use wheelchairs also have disabilities affecting their hands. You need to test out the extent to which people can grasp and hold things securely. This is

especially important when using electrical equipment or containers with hot contents, where there might be risk attached. At this point it is helpful to check the skills you identified next to each of the stages you identified earlier.

Where someone relies on help to carry out a part of the activity, it is important to determine the correct level of support, so that care staff give the right amount of help. It is all too easy to help too much, cheating the person out of the experience, or too little so that they are set up to fail and have a bad experience of participating.

These units of help we call prompts. Prompts fall basically into four categories:

Demonstration: Showing the client how to do a part or the whole of the task.

Verbal: Giving a verbal instruction, for example "Take the laundry out of the basket and put it on the floor".

Gesture: Giving an action instruction, for example pointing to the plates on the draining board and then pointing to the sink as an indication that the plates need to be put in the sink. This type of assistance is especially important where someone has hearing or language difficulties, or where they need additional cues to supplement verbal information.

Physical: This involves physically moving a person's limbs in order for them to carry out the task. For example you may need to hold a person's hand to operate a Compact Disc player.

In order to test the level of support needed, you will need to guide the person through the task in the following way:

Introduce the person to the task. For example, "We're now going to do the laundry. Let's go to the kitchen".

Wait to see if the person takes the initiative to start the task. If not, demonstrate the first stage.

From then on go down the list of prompts in the order described above:

SHOW – TELL – POINT – GUIDE

Make notes of the types of assistance the person required. They may need one or a combination of prompts. In this process you will need to consider: do they respond more often when you show them what needs doing rather than just tell them?

Let's now take the example of Nigel:
Nigel is 27 years old; he gets around in his wheelchair but depends on someone pushing it for him. He needs a body mould in the wheelchair to support him, relieve the pressure, and provide some comfort. He has some movement of his hands and arms although his grip is not strong. A member of the care staff did the washing with him and recorded all stages as on the chart opposite.

You could make a chart like this for common household tasks you do with people - it can be useful for other staff so that they can be consistent in involving the person when you are not there.

6. Carrying out the task: giving the level of help needed
Participation involves a balance between the person doing an activity and staff helping them, the constant factor being attention to the activity until it is done. It is a two way process which does not necessarily rely on words, but can also include actions. For staff it can be challenging, absorbing and hard work.

Reminders

• Always ensure that the person has full view and/or space to carry out the activity. Don't block their view by standing in front of them or reaching across them.

• Give clear instructions which have enough information in them to maximise action. Telling someone to "Put that in the thingy" or shouting from the other side of the room "Over there" gives the person very little information on which to base their next action.

• Where the person can carry out a stage independently and there is a lot of it to do, then there is the possibility of you sharing that stage by doing the work alongside them, for example, stripping a wall for re-papering or folding laundry. But otherwise you should stand back and be glad the person has something they can do which will use their time enjoyably.

Organisation

In order to assist people to participate in the activities of day-to-day living, there are two major areas of organisation to be attended to. They are:

1. Organising staff, and
2. Organising the person's time.

Your systems should ensure that there are care staff available in the right place at the right time for the activities you have chosen together to take place.

1. Organising staff

In order to do their work well, care staff need a set of flexible guidelines which

Stage of task	Nigel's skills	Assistance needed
1. Sorting the washing.	Is able to sort by colour and is able to unload dirty laundry basket at a slow pace.	The care staff member needs to hold the dirty laundry basket at waist height so that Nigel can reach the laundry.
2. Loading the washing machine.	Is unable to load washing machine due to the height of the machine door. Can push the door to close but not able to lock it.	Staff load the machine. He can push the door with a gestural and verbal prompt and with physical assistance lock the door.
3. Pouring the washing powder.	Unsteady hand in pouring.	Physical prompt required to pour the washing powder. He can slide the dispenser back with a gestural prompt.
4. Setting and starting the machine	Unable to identify numbers. Unable to grip and move dial to select wash.	Staff need to select wash and with a physical prompt he can start the cycle.
.5. Unloading the machine.	Unable to unload because machine too low.	Staff need to unload the machine.
6. Folding clean laundry ready for ironing.	Can fold small items.	Staff need to assist physically with large items in conjunction with a third person.

outline their responsibilities and inform them who does what with whom and at what time. The vehicles for planning this are the staff rota and daily shift planning, and the forum where they are planned should be regular staff meetings where arrangements can be drawn up to be confirmed in detail at the start of each shift. Time should be allowed at the staff meetings to cope with the dilemmas which arise on a regular basis, such as:

• What happens when there are too few staff on duty?

• How will you organise group participation?

• How do you divide your time so that people can participate?

• How do you decide which member of staff is doing what with whom?

• How do you ensure staff are on duty when you most need them, for example more at mealtimes and in the evenings when people might like to go out?

2. Organising activity

This essentially involves mapping out a daily and a weekly routine which takes into consideration each individual and their needs, and the household and its needs, and distributes these necessary activities throughout the day and week.

It might take the form of a house "diary" or wall planner, which includes regular things like shopping and washing alongside special things like doctors' appointments.

Once this is in place, your commitment to participation and the skills you develop in helping people has the best chance of success. Remember, participation does not just happen, you make it happen!

Points to remember

1. Participation means actively taking part.
2. It is about sharing activities which are generated through day-to-day living and finding tasks which are appropriate to individuals.
3. Participation is doing things **with** people, not for them.
4. It relies on the opportunities care staff create.
5. Opportunities for participation need to be identified and planned.
6. Activities need to be broken down into stages.
7. Individuals' abilities in carrying out the task need to be assessed.
8. The amount and nature of help given needs to be tried out and decided on.
9. **Everyone** is capable of participating.
10. People's involvement should be determined by their needs, likes, dislikes, choices and abilities.

References

1. The "Keeping Track" form is adapted from the Participation Index described in Developing Staffed Housing for People with Mental Handicaps, Mansell et al (1987) and is reprinted with permission from the teaching pack *Participation in Everyday Activities* in the Bringing People Back Home Series, Outset Publishing, Unit 8, Conqueror Industrial Estate, Moorhurst Road, St Leonards-on-Sea, East Sussex TN38 9NA.

Resources

Brown H, and Bailey R (1987). *Participation in Everyday Activities* – video assisted training pack in the Bringing People Back Home series, available from Outset Publishing (address above).

CHAPTER 9
Teaching new skills

Liz Garnham Hooper

• The principles of good teaching • Choosing which new skill to teach an individual • Preparation – setting goals, analysing the task, keeping records • How to teach – demonstration, prompts, gestures • Working with groups • What to do when things go wrong • Overcoming lack of motivation

A skill can be defined as "an ability acquired by training". In the support of people with severe learning disabilities, a skill can relate to the successful completion of a task at home, at work, any area of daily life. The approaches described can be used to teach absolutely new skills, or to increase an individual's ability at a task where they can already do part of it.

I have included some theory and "reasons for" teaching, as well as practical information about how to do it. The information given draws on Systematic Instruction[1] as well as other teaching systems, common sense and a lot of personal experience.

Principles

There are a number of principles which are present to a lesser or greater extent in most successful skills teaching programmes. Keeping them in mind will assist in decision-making and problem-solving, guiding our actions so that respect for the individual person is maintained and enhanced throughout the process. Where there is respect and appreciation for each person as an individual, they are much more likely to learn.

1. Whose responsibility? Very often the responsibility for learning a new task is placed solely on the shoulders of the person with learning disabilities, and a failure to learn is put down solely to lack of ability. We need to relieve people of that responsibility and take it on ourselves, so it is **our** responsibility to teach the person a given skill and if the person is not learning the fault lies with us: our way of teaching needs to change to help them learn.

2. Don't exclude: We have to believe that everybody can learn something, and bring optimism to our work. People with severe learning disabilities can and do learn complex skills, in their own time with good teaching; often achieving a greater success than we believed possible.

This does not mean you can teach anyone to do anything; the message is to broaden your horizons when considering people and what they want or need to learn. Be very wary of excluding people from opportunities to learn because you think their disability is too great to learn that task or activity. Think instead about *what it would take* to teach them or support them while they learn. In these circumstances we need to change the level of support, not the task or the person.

71

3. Balanced relationships: For the purposes of skills teaching, the only difference between you and the person with learning disabilities is that you know how to do the task and they do not. The object of the process therefore is for you to pass that on in an understandable way. In all other ways you are equal and joint partners in the process of learning. For while the individual will learn the task, you will learn much about them and your abilities as a teacher.

4. Being natural: Within this text the word natural will occur several times. By it I mean to emphasise what is ordinary, or what a non-disabled person would usually do. In making what we do as natural as possible, people are less stigmatised for being different. If we teach people to do something in the same way as everyone else, then in doing it they are visibly equal to non-disabled people, and will be more easily accepted by the community.

We have to consider too, what messages our behaviour sends out to other people about the individual we are with, and try to employ teaching methods which are discreet and yet get the job done. Naturalness has to be balanced with the inescapable fact that people with learning disabilities do sometimes need assistance which can look unnatural, for example helping someone count money in a shop. (How can we do that? Always aim for the least conspicuous way, and try not to interfere with the transaction between the individual and the shop keeper.)

5. Simplest is best: This principle does not deny that teaching skills to people with learning disabilities is often hard work, needing a lot of thought, planning and perseverance. It does mean that the end result needs to feel simple, uncluttered and as relaxed as possible; it is then more likely to happen and have a positive outcome for the individual. Often

time is limited, so why complicate matters unnecessarily with additional information or equipment? Do you really need to know how a camera works to take a photo?

6. Where to teach: The last and simplest principle is that you need to teach the skill where it will be performed: so teach shopping in a shop, dressing in the bedroom, cooking in the person's kitchen, teach money skills by having people use, handle and keep their own money.

Why teach skills?

We can assume that people with learning disabilities are provided with enough support to carry out daily life either by having difficult tasks completed for them or being allowed to participate with help and support. We need to justify why as care workers we want to take the extra time and effort involved in teaching people to do things for themselves. The Five Accomplishments[2] is a good framework in which to do this:

Presence

If someone is taught how to use a community facility – shop, library, pub – they are less dependent on staff time allowing them to use the facility. Therefore they are likely to use it more frequently and increase the times they are seen in the local community.

Participation

If someone uses a community facility themselves, the person will have more direct contact with the public, making relationships and becoming known in the local community. Work skills will open doors to participation in the work force as an equal citizen, with chances to form new relationships and improve social life.

Competence

The more skills someone learns, the greater the number of competences they have at their disposal. They are more likely to be seen as a skilled individual, rather than handicapped and dependent.

Choice
If someone can complete a task independently, they have some control over what to do and when, and rely less on staff time and inclination. They may also be able to choose between activities.

Dignity and respect
Being perceived as a competent individual will enhance the respect offered by other people: workers, family and the public. The person will also gain in self-respect and self-esteem. If a person learns more self-care skills, personal dignity and privacy are improved.

For care workers there is much satisfaction to be gained in teaching people new skills. We can feel that we are making a positive and practical contribution to an individual's quality of life.

What to teach

Where there are individual planning systems in services, these will guide workers directly or indirectly to skills the individual is or should currently be learning. However, not all plans have clearly defined goals which lead to skills teaching programmes. In their absence, where do you start? If this is the first time a skills teaching programme has been introduced to the individual, then the task needs to be selected with care by the person and yourself. The following factors will help you start:

• What does the individual want to do?

• What motivates this person? If this is not clear you have to use the smallest clues about their likes and dislikes. Do they like the smell of cooking, or noises when appliances are running?

• The task should meet a real need the individual has, not an artificial one. Don't try to teach someone to do puzzles, when they don't like doing puzzles.

• Teach a concrete task where there is a clear purpose so the person can understand what is being asked of them and it soon becomes obvious why. For example, it is difficult to teach people to sit down; easier to teach them to sit down and use a sewing machine, where it is clearer why you need to sit.

• Build on the person's strengths and preferences. For example, he can use switches and likes noise, so teach him how to use a blender to make soups, shakes etc.

• Consider physical capabilities. If the person uses a wheelchair, consider accessibility to buildings, the room, reaching necessary items from cupboards. (Ways of coping with additional difficulties will be dealt with below.)

• How old is the individual? Is this activity appropriate for their age?

• What sort of environment does the individual enjoy: noisy, quiet, lots of people, where there is space to move around, where there is music, or do they prefer to be away from distractions?

When you set out to teach someone something, ask yourself these questions:

• Can **you** do the task? If not you will need to learn it thoroughly first.

• Do you **believe** the person can learn the task? If you are confident, that will communicate itself to the user in a positive way. Alternatively if you begin thinking that the programme will fail, the person's task is made that much more difficult.

• How many teachers may be involved in teaching the task? Will they all co-operate and show enthusiasm? At first you may want to select a task where only one, two or three workers will be involved in the teaching, so you can closely monitor and learn as you go along.

You will also need to check these things out:

• **Time:** Will you have the necessary time? Whom do you need to talk to, to safeguard that time?

• **Frequency:** Ordinarily how often does the task need to be done? Those which occur more frequently, daily or twice a day, or a repetitive task, are easier to teach. This does not exclude weekly events, they are just more difficult and take longer.

• **Disturbances:** Try to pick a time when you are unlikely to be interrupted or called away. Can you arrange for other people to be occupied elsewhere?

• **"Props":** Can you ensure that what you need will be there – bread for making toast, bus pass for teaching independent travelling, etc?

• **Risk:** If there is a risk involved – crossing a road for example – is there a service policy to follow? Have the person's family and your managers been involved in the decision and agreed that it is worth taking the risk to gain the rewards?

• **Opportunity:** Will the person have the chance to use the skill when learned?

Hardly ever do we have perfect or near perfect conditions in which to teach; there will always be problems. We need to make the best of it but always work to improve the situation, rather than waiting for someone else to change it.

Setting goals

Once you have decided what kind of thing you will be teaching you need to set a clear, defined goal: one that everyone has agreed to (or as many people as you can persuade).

One area commonly used to begin to teach new skills or extend existing skills is cooking. People with learning disabilities often have "learn to cook more independently" as a goal on their individual plans. However, this is too global; it needs to be broken down to a more specific target skill. "Learn to make and butter toast" or "Learn to use the oven", for example. The latter are much clearer and you will also know when you have achieved them.

When setting goals, it may be necessary to give a certain time limit by which the skill will have been learned by the individual. This can be useful as it spurs people into action and you will have a date when the programme will be evaluated. However, if it is used to prove or disprove an individual's ability to learn, then it is counterproductive and should be avoided. Setting such a date is a skill in itself, often acquired through experience. You need to consider the variables:

- how often the opportunity for "practice" will occur
- the complexity of the skill
- the current abilities of the person with learning disabilities
- the teaching abilities of the teachers
- the motivation of the person to learn the skill
- how many people are teaching, and how consistent they are.

Task analysis

Now the goal has been agreed, the next activity is for the service workers to complete the task analysis. This can often seem a pointless time-consuming activity, especially for everyday tasks which "everybody" knows how to do. It also rarely involves people with learning disabilities, so we need to take time away from direct work, and be able to justify why.

Task analysis can be defined as the

breaking down of a task into a number of sequential steps which are written down. Common examples of task analyses are recipes, or assembly instructions for DIY furniture.

Why is task analysis useful?
• There may be a number of different ways a certain task can be done. For example making tea: do you get the cups out as the kettle is boiling, or do you get everything ready and then boil the water? You and your colleagues will have to decide a "team" order which everyone sticks to, thus promoting consistency and better teaching.

• As the steps of a task are identified it is easier to teach and to recognise when the individual will need more help.

• Completing a task analysis will help you decide how to teach a task, and this information can be shared with others.

• Without a task analysis, accurate record keeping is practically impossible.

A question often asked is "How many steps should the task be broken down to?" Again it is an individualised process, depending on the task and the individual. But there are some general guidelines which can be observed:

To begin with, divide the task into the steps any average person would need; each new step begins at a point where you would need to give Mr or Ms Average more information in order to complete the next part of the task. We start like this as it assumes that the individual can learn at a natural rate, and we should only move away from that plan when an individual is having difficulties. If from our knowledge of the individual we know they will have difficulty with certain parts, then we make the steps smaller at that point. You do not need to break the whole task down into minute steps.

The following is an example of "Making Tea" using "Mr or Ms Average" steps and tiny steps.

Example 1
1. Fill the kettle with water.
2. Switch on and boil the water.
3. Put 2 teabags in the teapot.
4. Pour milk into the mugs.
5. Pour boiled water onto the teabags.
6. Pour the tea onto the milk.
7. Offer sugar to others and help self.
8. Drink tea.

Example 2
1. Place right hand on kettle lead where it plugs into the kettle and grip firmly.
2. Steady kettle with left hand on handle.
3. Pull out lead from kettle with right hand and release.
4. Take lid off kettle with right hand.
5. Let go of the kettle handle with left hand.
6. Pick up kettle with right hand.
7. Carry kettle to the sink.
8. Position kettle under the cold tap.

As you can see, in Example 2 it is going to take many more steps to arrive at a mug of tea. It will take a long time to write it all down and may be difficult to learn. Example 1 may be all you need for the individual you are working with. You may only need to elaborate steps 1 and 2; many people already know steps 6, 7 and 8, so they need little if any further work.

How to complete a task analysis
1. Decide at what point the task begins and ends: for example with tea making, does the individual start by gathering everything together, or will you do that and the task begin with filling the kettle? When does shopping end: when you leave the shop, when you arrive home, when you take your coat off, or when the shopping is put away?
2. Watch someone who is good at it, doing the task several times in their natural setting. This will help you form a visual

image of the task. Don't try and think about it from the office, you'll miss something out.

3. Check the task analysis by asking someone else to follow it exactly. Does it accurately describe everything that needs to be done?

4. Make sure anyone who is teaching has seen the analysis thoroughly and agrees to use it as a blueprint even if they usually do things differently.

The task analysis is for *your* information. it is **not** designed to be given to the person with learning disabilities as a set of instructions.

Natural cues

In any task there are a number of features that are constant and will provide the learner with cues as to their next action, regardless of whether you are there or not. We all use natural cues of the time, but we are mostly unaware that we use them.

For example, when you walk into a place selling food, how do you know whether to walk to the counter and order or sit at a table? Queues of people, the pay till and displays of available food are the cues in a "fast food" place; menus on the table and people hovering to seat and serve you give another message.

Natural cues are unique to each situation and can only be found by going there and having a go. The cues need to be identified and taught to the learner. Natural cues are also available in everyday tasks: for example there are different colour tap tops for hot and cold; most automatic kettles click when they switch off, informing the learner to pour the water on to the tea.

Seeking out natural cues is part of good preparation, and should be done with the task analysis. Note which cues the learner takes notice of and cue them accordingly. Consistency is important, so all teachers should use the same cues for each step.

Deafness and blindness: Apart from the obvious points – not using gesture when a person is unable to see well, or verbal cues for someone who does not hear well – the teacher needs to make increased efforts to point out the natural cues that indicate a step is complete. When planning sessions, consider how information will best be understood by the learner.

Record keeping

This activity can also be known as data collection, and it is often an unpopular activity. Records are seldom well used, even when they have been well kept, so let us be clear about why you need to bother, what to keep in the file and how to do it.

Why keep records

1. You need accurate information on how the individual's learning is progressing.

2. You need to know when the individual has learned the skill, and completed it correctly several times in a row, so you can leave them in future to do it alone.

3. To help make teaching decisions. For example if a person continues to find a particular step difficult, when they have learned the rest. This is especially important when different teachers are involved who may not notice small improvements.

4. If a teacher is away or has not completed a session for a few days, they can see what is happening straight away.

5. If learning is slow to progress, then being able to demonstrate it is happening, maintains everyone's motivation.

6. The individual is trusting you to do a good job, and keeping accurate records is part of that job.

7. Where risk is involved, you will be able to show that the person has learned the skill safely.

How to do it

You need to set out a recording sheet, with an abbreviated form of each step in the

STEPS	Number of times taught (dates)											
	12/1	14/1	15/1	22/1	26/1	31/1	2/2	4/2	5/2	9/2	12/2	15/2
1. Sort dirty clothing	✗	✗	✗	✗	✗	✗	✗	✗	✗	✗	✓	✓
2. Carry to utility room	✗	✗	✗	✓	✓	✓	✓	✓	✓	✓	✓	✓
3. Place clothes in machine	✗	✗	✗	✗	✗	✓	✓	✓	✓	✓	✓	✓
4. Fill powder dispenser	✓	✓	✓	✓	✓	✓	✓	✓	✓	✓	✓	✓
...and so on...												

Learner: Caroline B   Task: Personal Laundry   Teachers: Anne, Sam

Keeping records is unpopular but important, as it helps everyone see what progress is made.

task analysis corresponding to a series of blank squares, which can be filled in during or after teaching. For example, "Doing personal laundry".

The Task Analysis might read:
Step 1. Empty the laundry bin and sort the clothes into two separate heaps, one for whites and one for colours.
Step 2. Gather up the whites and carry them downstairs to the utility room.
Step 3. Open the washing machine door and put the clothes inside.
Step 4. Find washing powder and scoop, measure out the correct amount of powder into the right compartment of the dispenser...*and so on.*
The Data Sheet for this might be a chart like the one above.

Now you can see there is an opportunity to record how the individual performed each step of the task, over a number of opportunities they had to learn it.
The simplest way to record performance is with an agreed coding system, such as:

✓ - the individual performed the step without any assistance from the teacher.

✗ - the individual needed some help.

Remembering the principle "Simplest is Best", we only need to keep one sort of information: either ✗ – what a person does with help, or ✓ – what they do without help.

Early on in teaching it is easiest to remember those steps the individual completed independently, because there will be fewer of those at the beginning. You can focus on remembering where you didn't need to give help and tick the sheet at the end of the session.

Later on, as the person has learned much of the task, you can switch the system and remember the ✗s where the person did need assistance; at that stage of teaching this will be the least amount of information for you to remember. If the task is too long to remember all steps accurately, record some at a natural break during the task.

If the task being taught is something which repeats itself frequently, you can consider keeping records at intervals, eg every fifth time the individual washes their hands. This will be less intensive on teaching, reduce the volume of records and still provide you with the necessary information. Remember to note on the record sheet if you are keeping these kinds of records.

When keeping records of skills teaching there are a few points to note:
1. Be honest. It is often tempting to put a ✓when you really did provide some,

although small, piece of help. We all want to give credit especially if the individual is making huge efforts. However, it will not help them in the long term and could lead to mistakes later on. This is particularly important if you are teaching something risky like crossing the road.

2. Avoid being "fuzzy". Don't put a half tick if they did most of the step right and only needed a prompt to complete it.

3. Concentrate – especially when the individual has almost learned the skill, often a time when sloppiness and over-confidence lead to mistakes.

How to teach

Up to this point the teacher and learner have not come together in the teaching situation, the work has been preparatory. Good preparation, though it seems laborious, is always worthwhile and should not be shortened in the interests of speed. With time and practice you will find it easier and become faster at it. At this point you should be able to complete the task without thinking, so you can concentrate on the learner, and not be thinking about what they need to do next at each point.

Now you are ready to teach, How? At the beginning I said that skills teaching is passing information from yourself to the learner in a way they can understand. There are three basic principles to that:

1. When to give information.
2. What kind of information to give.
3. How much information to give at any one time.

WHEN
The individual will learn by actually doing the task as it should be done: they need to get into a rhythm and routine of "doing the task right". By implication this means that early on in teaching, the teacher does not allow the learner to make any mistakes (this is called "errorless learning"). The teacher must be on hand to anticipate and prevent errors.

At the beginning of the programme, the teacher needs to give the learner enough information to complete each step correctly, just as they are about to begin performing the necessary movements. If the learner is about to pick up an item, the teacher is very positive in directing them towards the correct one and ensuring a good grip.

As the teaching sessions progress the teacher can wait a little and allow the learner to demonstrate whether they know which item to pick up, only intervening if the learner is about to pick up the wrong one or looks as if they might drop it. Again the intervention is positive: giving information about which is the correct item, not saying "no" as it creates a nega-tive atmosphere and learners perform best in positive learning situations.

If the teacher misjudges and the learner picks up a wrong item, the fault lies with the teacher for not spotting and preventing an imminent mistake. The teacher should apologise and correct the mistake themselves.

When the person can more or less do the task, when the teacher believes and the records show that the learner can do much of the task without help, then the teacher may give the learner the opportunity to correct their own mistakes (this is called self-correction). If however the learner carries on and didn't notice the mistake, then again it is the teacher who has misjudged the learner's capabilities to do the task independently.

Giving information

The question of when to give information is individualised in the way described above, according to the learner and the situation. Generally speaking, we give positive information to the learner, correcting mistakes before they happen.

There are a number of ways of giving people information, which can be called a variety of names: cues, prompts, assists, etc. I have chosen to use prompts as I think it is the most familiar term.

DEMONSTRATION (showing the person): This can be used to give the learner the idea of what the task looks like as it is going to be taught (especially important if it is an unfamiliar task), and what (if appropriate) the end product looks like. Some individuals may give more attention to a demonstration than others; some people do not like to or cannot watch and want to be involved straight away, which is fine. Other people may like a demonstration at the beginning of each session and gain a lot of information from it.

PHYSICAL PROMPTS (guiding the person by touch): These are often very specific movements such as manipulating the hands for a particular part of the task. It is a simple way of giving complex information: think how much easier it is to physically help someone unscrew a jar lid than to try and explain how to do it.

Later on, physical prompts can be non-specific, such as a gentle nudge in the right direction or a touch on the hand to indicate which hand holds an item.

GESTURES (pointing in the right direction) Sometimes you can do a "demonstration in the air" of the way in which the learner should manipulate that part of the task. Again, it can be used to give complex information in a simple and clear way. Gestures can be either very specific, with the finger very close to the next item to be used, or vague waves towards what the person should be working on next. They are extremely useful and easy for people to understand,

providing the learner can see them. Obviously they are not very useful for people who have a significant visual impairment.

VERBAL PROMPTS (telling the person) These are extremely useful when used correctly, but people tend to give too many verbal instructions and use language which is too complicated (see Chapter 5). **Any** spoken words during the teaching of a task should be about the task and give information to the learner about what to do next; everything else is superfluous and merely clutters teaching, distracting both parties from focusing on the job to be done.

The closest analogy one can make is to imagine that on your first driving lesson, your instructor carried on a conversation with you about your holiday, while teaching you to drive! Driving instructors generally provide us with a good role model of uncluttered, task-focused verbal instruction.

Verbal prompts can be very specific – "Pick up the spoon", "Turn on the tap" – or later on in teaching when less help is needed, "What happens next?". This is not to say we never have a conversation, but that we distinguish task-focused teaching time, from conversational time which could occur at the end of a session. People with learning disabilities pick up clues from our tone of voice, so change it slightly, to sound business-like but not authoritarian, when involved in teaching.

People whose behaviour we find challenging may not need special considerations other than particular attention paid to selection of the task, focusing on the task, and redirection back to the task.

However, lack of concentration is often mentioned. Be prepared to be flexible and allow people time away from the task for a few minutes, before directing them back. Do not, for example, insist that people sit down to complete table top skills. The important issue is engagement with the task; sitting down may well occur naturally later on. Be prepared for the behaviours to occur and have planned strategies of how you will deal with them. For example if someone rips a shirt does it mean the session ends, or do you find another shirt and then continue? Seek the advice of others (and see Chapter 7).

Partial assistance

There are some people who no matter how good the teaching will always need some help to carry out particular tasks. This means we should plan for continual ongoing assistance, for example in travelling to a facility, but teach as much of the task as we can to the individual: using the facility once there, paying for themselves, knowing their way around, and so on.

Avoid distractions

When teaching we traditionally tend to use a lot of positive reinforcement, especially in the form of verbal praise, believing it necessary in order that the person continues to be motivated to do the task. However, if we are paying proper attention and the individual is learning something that they want to do, much of it is unnecessary and patronising. This sort of positive reinforcement is saying "I'll let you know when you do something right" and thus the individual becomes dependant on that positive approval.

We should substantially decrease our verbal praise to a more natural level, and so allow the learner to rely on their own sense of knowing when they are doing it right. Marc Gold called this strategy "No News is Good News": the teacher says "If I am not interfering with you and the task then everything is going well". Thus people do not become dependant on

positive approval from the teacher after each step. We do still offer praise, but more naturally, for instance when the task is completed or the learner has worked particularly hard.

This is a difficult strategy at first because we are conditioned into saying "Well done" and "Good" every time the person does something right. People with learning disabilities are also used to us saying it and have to learn the new way of working. However, if you try it you will see that they can do without constant fussing and prefer more adult appreciation.

It is also important to look at what the person is doing and not encourage unnecessary eye contact. How can we expect people to concentrate if we are not showing them how by concentrating on what is going on ourselves? Do not encourage the learner to look at your face – you want them to look at the work they are doing.

If the person starts distracting behaviour such as finger flicking, gazing round the room, constant chatter, try to ignore non-task behaviour (unless the person is very distressed), and gently re-focus their attention on the task by providing a prompt for the next step.

Do not tell the person off on these occasions, rather model and encourage good concentration skills. If you become involved in the non-task behaviour, the session's focus will shift from learning a task to controlling behaviour, and it will take much longer to re-focus the learner on the task.

How much information?

The teacher should make a conscious effort to fade out of the learning situation, and not become an artificial part of it. Throughout the teaching you must be aware of how much prompting is being given, and keep it to the minimum amount necessary for the learner to complete the task correctly. The teacher should try to give less assistance at that particular step than they did during the previous session. When the learner is at a part of the task where they are competent the teacher should physically move away, only coming in close again at a step where more assistance is needed. Also *within* a step there is room to fade – from a specific gesture to one which is slightly vague.

Aids to learning

There may be instances when you need to give some kind of specialised help to a learner, when they are getting stuck on part of a task because of their particular disability.

Special aids should only be added as a last resort, or to overcome a specific difficulty, but they can be helpful. For example you can help people to recognise bus numbers by giving them a card with a number on to match up to that on the front of the bus.

Working with groups

So far I have been talking about skills teaching on the ratio of one teacher to one learner, which is more achievable in some services than others. It is the most effective way to teach and worth organising time to do. However, if you are responsible for a group and unable to get away there are some things you can still teach in a structured way:

• You can set most group members up with some work they can do and concentrate on one person for several minutes, teaching one to one when they are at a part of the task they find particularly difficult.

• You can have selected tasks which the same group members work on consistently, thus providing opportunity

for learning, for example tea making.

• You can all be doing the same activity and learn at the same rate; this can be frustrating for some of the group and humiliating for others unless handled very sensitively.

• If there are two workers it is easier, as one worker can manage the group for 30 minutes while the other offers one to one teaching time to one group member.

• You can manage the room so that you attend to people at frequent intervals, asking others to wait if they come to a part of the task they are unsure of.

Lack of motivation

Often we hear that people with learning disabilities are not motivated to learn; they are described as being "unable" to learn, or as lazy or stubborn. Often the real reason is that we are teaching people boring tasks. Learning many self-care activities – bathing, dressing, brushing teeth – is not highly motivating for many people, and these may not be the best targets for initial teaching programmes.

Teach something new and challenging to the person. If we have to teach something mundane can we offer more verbal praise, without being patronising? If getting dressed is the task, can we have a favourite breakfast ready for the person to eat afterwards, or organise the family or care workers to show interest and offer compliments on the person's appearance?

Thus we can ensure that people receive additional encouragement, manipulating natural events into a rewarding sequence.

When things go wrong

What can you do?

• Review use of prompts; ask someone else to observe and comment.

• Do some steps need to be broken down further to pinpoint and resolve the difficulty?

• Do you need to introduce an aid, for example a photograph of the bus stop where the individual needs to get off?

• Has the learner lost their motivation? How can you build in more rewards?

• Is the learner bored with the task before they have learned it? If so you may need a break, or you may have to start again with something else.

• If the learner seems to make deliberate mistakes, perhaps they want you around for social reasons. Can you arrange a time for socialisation?

• How focused on the task are you? Have you been too distracted by other events so that the learner feels let down?

• Is it too long between teaching sessions? Can you increase the frequency?

In conclusion

It is impossible to be prescriptive about every task you may want to teach, or the characteristics of the individuals you are working with, but you should now have some ideas on how to get started and how to deal with some of the situations you may face. The best thing you can do is start somewhere and learn as you go along. Start with one person with learning disabilities and one task, and build on that.

Try to keep an open mind about who might learn what, and you will be pleasantly surprised. Remember that events rarely run smoothly, so be flexible and adaptable: don't give up at the first sign of trouble. Good luck!

Action plan

1. With the person with learning disabilities and other workers, select an area to work on and arrive at a specific goal of the skills teaching programme. Set a date to begin and a date to review progress.

2. Familiarise yourself with the task and the sequence of events within it; you need to be able to do it without thinking.

3. Construct a task analysis, making a mental note of the natural cues within it.

4. Draw up a recording sheet, and decide on the code to be used for recording.

5. Hold a meeting with possible other teachers. Ensure they know the task analysis, recording sheet and natural cues to be used. Highlight areas of possible inconsistency, and decide a common strategy.

6. Ensure you have the support necessary of others: managers, other workers, family.

7. Begin teaching, and keep accurate records, change cues etc. as necessary.

8. Evaluate progress as you go along, and with others on the agreed review date.

9. Celebrate success with the individual and other workers.

10. Once a skill has been taught, ensure the person has opportunities to use it.

11. What are you going to do next? Build on your success.

References

1. Systematic Instruction is compiled and developed by Dr Marc Gold and Marc Gold & Associates in the USA.

2. The Five Accomplishments (John O'Brien), see Chapter 1 pages 14-15.

CHAPTER 10

Day services: new opportunities

Aideen Jones and Jill Shepherd

• How day services have changed over the years • An alternative model: wider opportunities and more community contact • Individual programmes • Setting goals and keeping records of achievement

Day services is a term which covers an enormous range of provision for people with learning disabilities. Chapter 11 will discuss employment in detail, but we mention it here because we feel strongly that work experience and employment opportunities should always be considered as part of the "package" of day services open to people with learning disabilities. Work is one way in which we can find valued social roles among friends and colleagues and being paid is important too! All these things should be taken into account also for people we work with who rely on some form of day service.

Day centre, day care, adult training centre, workshop, work are all words you will hear to describe places people go to between 9 am and 5 pm. We are not only interested in where people go, however, but in what they do there.

An alternative model

Day services have been traditionally run from day centres where the building and overheads eat up a large amount of the total budget. We have been lucky enough in our area to be given our own day services budget, and we decided early on not to tie up the money in buildings, overheads and full-time staff. This is how we went about setting up the service:

• We recruited a co-ordinator who explored all the activities available in the local community.

• The co-ordinator met with residents and keyworkers to see what individual needs and interests were.

• The co-ordinator then matched up individual needs to activities and people who could support the resident in these activities.

• Every six months, needs are re-assessed.

This did not happen overnight, and sometimes things don't work out, but we have the flexibility to change when the need arises. We recruit sessional staff to support individual activities. Full-time members of staff are unlikely to be able to offer swimming, pottery, sewing, photography, driving, literacy skills and physiotherapy, so the use of sessional staff works well for the people with learning disabilities enrolled in the day service.

We try to use local facilities such as community centres, local swimming pools,

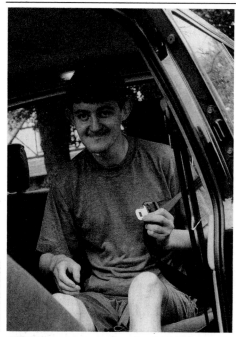

Photo: Sue Benson

Off for a swim: try to use local facilities and go in small numbers.

sports centres and adult education. Many of our activities are still separate sessions for "handicapped" people, but using facilities where there is a cafe or coffee bar allows some mixing and social contact with the public. Many of our residents are wheelchair users and we still face access problems in public buildings. Because we are trying to overcome this isolation of people with learning disabilities in the community our next stage of development will include establishing our own groups (including a music group) in public facilities (such as a community centre) involving one or two of our residents and then opening them to the public. A yoga group set up in this way has worked well.

Individual programmes

Most residents participate in six to eight different activities each week, with one day a week spent at home helping with domestic tasks. Individual group sessions,

small group activity and a few larger groups can be supported by up to one to one staffing. This is necessary because of the physical needs of the residents, and it improves the quality of the experience. We achieve this by using sessional staff, community service volunteers, and sometimes input from residential staff.

Creating opportunities

Before planning day activities for someone, it is important to get to know him or her. You cannot even guess at what kind of things they may enjoy until you have spent some time finding out what kind of person they are.

If you were invited to a party by a friend you might meet a wide range of people with varying interests: gardening, photography, motor bikes, ballroom dancing, and so on. When you meet a group of people with learning disabilities, they have interests which are just as wide ranging. It is possible that they have not had the chance to explore all their interests, or even to identify them in such a way that they can describe them in words. Your first task is to keep an open mind and try to understand the individual on their own terms. Learning disabilities do not prevent people from enjoying many experiences which are generally available, or from developing skills in many different areas of life.

Having got to know the person as an individual, and gained some ideas about what they might like to try, you have the problem of "starting where they are". This process may involve a lot of hard work and imagination. If they miss out essential steps in understanding and learning, they will never be able to make use of the opportunities that you provide.

Imagine you decided that a child would benefit from being able to read. If you gave them a novel without teaching them how to make sense of the words and sentences then their failure would be certain, and would not be their fault at all.

It is easy to set service users up to fail in this way, and a challenge to our skills and sensitivity to make sure that we avoid this failure by developing alongside the people that we support. It may be necessary to call in outside help at this point.

A young man who suffers from cerebral palsy had no means of communicating except by negative body language - refusing something by cringing into his wheelchair and grimacing. The staff team who support him needed the help of a specialist speech therapist to begin a process which could develop at the young man's pace, so that he can now signal when he needs help, and can choose between drinks, different foods and so on. We hope this will lead on to him making other choices of activities.

Creating opportunities does not depend on choosing activities from a list and allocating people to a programme. A quality service is provided by knowing the person as an individual, understanding their needs and preferences and building on their strengths, at a pace which they can cope with.

Planning activities

We all benefit from having reasonably balanced lifestyles, when we can. We need physical exercise, mental stimulation, social contact, emotional security and spirituality (which can come from religion, beauty, art, music or other sources). We also need to be busy sometimes and quiet at others; to be serious sometimes and have fun at others.

Because people have a wide range of interests and abilities, so we need to consider a range of needs when we help them to plan daytime activities.

Education is important for all of us. We may be studying a language at evening class, trying out new cookery recipes at home or having staff training sessions. People with learning disabilities may be learning to read, practising dressing themselves or understanding their environment by touching new shapes and textures.

Their lifestyles must also be (as described by the mother of an individual with learning disabilities) "more than just responding to basic needs". If we are creating a whole living environment for people, then the value of dozing in front of an old film on Sunday afternoon must be recognised alongside learning to swim on Monday morning. For a young man to go to a nightclub with others of his age is as important as teaching him to cross the road, if he is to develop as a balanced person who feels respected as an adult.

It is difficult for us to cope with the conflicts involved in planning activities for someone who is adult in years but may be childlike in some areas of their intellectual development. Dignity and respect in language and attitudes are vitally important especially if you need to make compromises, as for example when you feel that the best stimulus for someone may come from a child's toy or "junior" equipment.

It is possible, however, to choose toys without childish pictures and symbols, in primary colours rather than nursery pink and blue. If they are removed from the original boxes and always referred to as equipment that the person can work with, rather than toys to be played with, then they become just that, and the attitudes of others around will tend to follow the respectful lead.

Working together

There needs to be a very close working relationship between day and residential staff so that people's lives are not divided into two different areas, run by different people in different ways. A keyworker system can help to ensure that important information is passed on. You may hear people say that there needs to be a clear distinction between these two areas of a person's life, but it can be confusing for people with learning disabilities if the goalposts keep moving. We all need to feel that there is an overall pattern to our lives, which makes sense.

Joining in as equals

It is also important to find activities where everyone can participate equally, such as going swimming and listening to music. Almost everyone, whatever their level of learning or physical disability, can enjoy being in water. Differences between levels of ability are much less important when everyone is in a swimming pool, just as when a group of people listen to music, enjoy looking at paintings or participate in a religious activity. Who can say which member of a concert audience is enjoying the music most?

So a programme of activities needs to be balanced, and to be based on what you know of the person's needs and preferences. It is likely to involve some education, whether in class or informally at home. It should also include some physical exercise, a good amount of fun and relaxation, and space for being alone and doing whatever seems to be a good idea at the time.

Community resources

If people with learning disabilities are to use their community to the full, it is important to find out what is available. This takes time. You will know about some aspects of your community but you will need to ask people about other things. Things like swimming pools and cinemas are fairly easy, but a club for pigeon fanciers or a drop-in art class may be less well advertised. Find out from colleagues, friends, local newspapers and so on. Libraries and the Citizens Advice Bureau are good sources of information.

Ask other staff where they go socially and what interests they have. It may be possible to tie up with these.

> One young man is accompanied on outings to the local nightclubs by a member of staff who enjoys "clubbing". She is happy to arrange her hours round a visit to the club every few weeks, and suggested that he take a nap in the afternoon (as she does) so that he can enjoy the evening without getting too tired.

You may find that a bit of imagination is needed for people to enjoy some facilities. A woman who plays indoor bowls from a wheelchair uses a short length of plastic guttering to set the bowls on course.The local tenpin bowling alley has inflatable "sausages" that fill the gutters, so success in hitting the skittles is guaranteed.

> A swimming pool with graduated sloping access rather than steps, has fitted a plastic garden chair with wheels so that wheelchair users can enter the water in a dignified way.

Ask managers – especially those of council-run facilities – what they can do to make access easier for the people you support. Point out that they can often obtain grants from local authorities and charities to help with the cost.

A big obstacle when using community facilities is that of public prejudice. We have to admit to this, try to find ways to cope with it and change people's attitudes. To ignore it often leads to confrontation and a lot of embarrassment and hurt for people with learning disabilities.

The first line of attack is for us, as care staff, to help the people we support to fit into the community. This involves basic practical steps to avoid them being seen as different:

• As far as possible, go into the community in very small groups rather than in large numbers.

• Make sure that everyone is properly equipped for what they are doing; this helps them to look competent and be taken seriously. They should have the right type of clothing for the activity – a properly fitting swimsuit and an adult towel, for instance, not one with a cartoon or child's motif.

• They should carry their own membership card for entry, and a purse or wallet with the right money for a drink. They can hand over, say, £1, and know that they will get change, rather than holding out a purse for the till assistant to take what is needed.

These types of practical details can transform "the mentally handicapped group" at the local swimming pool into ordinary members of the public using a community resource, even if they do need some help and support to do so.

If you need to obtain support from community groups, make contact with them before taking people with learning disabilities to new places. Explain who you are and what you want. Understand the concerns of people who, for instance, may not know how to respond to someone who does not speak.

Try to keep a balance between insisting on the rights of people with learning disabilities, and helping people in the community to become involved gently, at a pace that they can accept.

This is difficult work, and you may well need support from your colleagues.

Remember how much the people you support will gain from your efforts. It will easily outweigh the efforts you put in.

Keeping records

It is not essential to keep endless A4 files of every aspect of day service provision. As an aid to communication and to give the person a sense of history, we suggest the following:

• Have a list of the goals for each activity. A goal does not have to be complex – the goal for swimming might be a) to have fun, and b) to use leg muscles in the water.

• Evaluate each activity once a month, making minor changes where necessary.

• Re-write the goals at six monthly reviews.

• Have a weekly timetable in the person's diary.

• Use photographs, audio tapes and video tape to keep a record of what the person is achieving, and let them show these at their individual planning review (see Chapter 4) so that everyone can share in their achievements.

Points to remember

1. Work **with** the person, not for them.
2. Services must be individual – everyone is different.
3. Dignity and respect must be maintained whatever you are doing.
4. There is always a way to communicate: keep looking.
5. Be creative – don't be limited by what has happened in the past.
6. Continually ask "Why?" and "What's it for?"
7. Be part of your community.
8. Challenge the local community to join you.
9. Make things as "ordinary" as possible.
10. Don't forget time for doing nothing.

CHAPTER 11

Finding and keeping a job

Mike Crowhurst, Liz Henderson, Penelope Ledger

• The right to employment • Everyone can do a job • Sheltered employment or supported employment • Work experience • Looking for a job • Motivation and support • Benefits explained • Sources of help

People with learning disabilities have the same right to employment opportunities as you and I. This statement and belief is fundamental to the philosophy of *an ordinary life* which provides the foundation on which most of today's services are based. We in services are good at making noble and "right-on" statements about employment and other issues, but services in general have a poor record in finding meaningful employment for people with learning disabilities, and supporting them through the process.

If the philosophy of an ordinary life could be summed up in one sentence, then it would be that people with learning disabilities should be given access to at least all the opportunities that you and I have, living as part of a community. This is not just about treating people equally, it's about redressing the balance for people who have been treated badly by society, as well as having difficulties of their own, and offering them support to compete on an equal basis with everyone else.

If we acknowledge that people with learning disabilities are as much like us as not, then we need only look at our own lives to see the wealth of experience that employment offers:

• A chance to work with others who are non-disabled;

• something to talk about: what is the first thing that you usually ask someone when you meet them for the first time – "So what do you do for a living then?"

• self esteem and status;

• the opportunity to be a contributing member of your community, to contribute to other's lives;

• the opportunity to make friends and acquaintances;

• an introduction into groups of people who have similar skills or hobbies;

• the opportunity to earn your own money, which you can spend on yourself, or on whatever you like.

• Employment is a valued element in the lifestyle of most people, with or without a learning disability. Think how much time you spend at work.

Breaking down myths

The biggest obstacle for people with learning disabilities is not lack of skills, it is lack of people believing in them. Even people with the most severe learning disabilities can work if they are given the right help.

Training in Systematic Instruction (TSI) is an intensive training method developed by Dr Marc Gold and Marc Gold and Associates in the USA. Using this method of teaching, people with the most severe learning difficulties have been taught to carry out complex and intricate tasks, such as the assembly of bike drum brakes and other production line assemblies. Structured teaching and on-the-job training is essential for people who may find it difficult to just "pick things up". Chapter 8 on teaching will help to set out the basics for teaching people with learning disabilities new work skills.

Work opportunities

There are essentially two types of employment opportunities:

1) Sheltered employment

This is by far the most common employment for people with learning disabilities in this country, and indeed in Europe. Sheltered employment workshops are usually found in Adult Training Centres (ATCs) or Social Education Centres. Often people work at these centres for many years under supervision, on low or even token pay, in a segregated environment. Relatively few people proceed to open employment, raising the question of whether the person is really a "trainee" or an employee. Are they in fact being "prepared" for anything other than retirement?

There are some good sheltered employment projects around, but they should be viewed only as short term, and as stepping stones to open employment. Remember, it is easy for an organisation to go through the motions of supporting people into employment, but would you

and I be content to do work for years with sometimes little or no variety, for a pittance of a wage, in a segregated environment?

2) Supported employment

Supported employment has been developed extensively in the United States over the last ten years. It works by placing someone with a learning disability in a suitable job, and providing them with training and any other additional support they need to get the job done. As the person becomes more skilled and competent within their new job, the support is gradually withdrawn.

Supported Employment has the advantage of giving the worker a real job in a real workplace. The worker works with the help of a job coach and perhaps other colleagues, and receives training specific to the job in hand. From the employer's point of view, they can rest assured that with the help of a job coach the job will be completed to the highest level. Experience in the United States and in this country has shown that many individuals formerly excluded from employment can and do prosper in a range of jobs.

Motivation

Many of the people we support have for most of their lives been denied the opportunity to make even the most basic and simple decisions about their lives. So making a decision about finding a job is an awesome prospect, and people will require an immense amount of support.

Part of our job in supporting people is to acknowledge the anxieties they face in this decision-making process. Many people have learned that it is easier to say no than to face the unknown, even if it means they are likely to spend hours being bored or frustrated as a result – it's a case of the devil you know. This is perhaps the biggest challenge, to find ways of supporting people through their anxieties, and encouraging and motivating them to make the first step. Remember your first interview; the first time you started a job.

Imagination is essential if we are to find work for people outside sheltered employment. Employers won't be queuing up to offer jobs, especially in these times of high unemployment. If you are serious, then do your homework:

• Find out a bit about a prospective employer, identify the job you think the person you support is interested in.

• Consider what is involved in training someone in the task.

• Consider how many days of the week the person wants to work, it could be part time or perhaps a job share.

• Talk to your organisation; be clear about how much staff resources it can commit to the project.

Experience tells us that most employers will listen to a good idea. When you have reached the stage of talking to a potential employer, it's down to you to sell the idea, so turn up prepared and well presented.

The next step

So far so good; your next step is to gather information about the individual to establish what kind of job might suit them. Parents or relatives could be involved if appropriate, to ensure all relevant information is included. They could also have useful contacts with local businesses which may be worth exploring.

A meeting should be held to compile a job search profile for the individual (see above). Try to think creatively. Concentrate on abilities rather than disabilities, while still acknowledging that there may be some areas of difficulty which could be a barrier to certain jobs.

JOB SEARCH PROFILE

The individual

• Sketch a plan of person's current daily activities, at home and out of the home.

• List the type of support the person currently requires with the above activities.

• Decide what kinds of support work well when teaching the person a new skill.

• Does the person currently work – include household tasks, work tasters, sheltered work and paid work.

• Consider any interests the person has in activities in and out of home.

The local area

• Find out what type of job opportunities exist.

• Public transport – what type is available and which places can be reached. What kind of support does the person need when using public transport?.

• What local resources are there? Is there a job centre, specialist employment service for people with learning disabilities, job club or training scheme the person could use?

To ensure that the individual is given the opportunity to get involved, plan ahead. Think about how you can support them in making their choice.

Suggestions

• Collect and use leaflets about different jobs from the local job centre or careers office.

• Use photos showing people doing some different jobs, collected from recruitment leaflets from larger companies, or magazines.

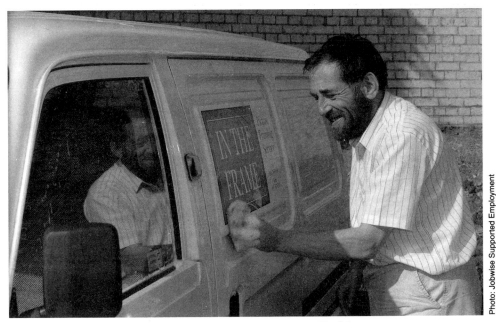

Photo: Jobwise Supported Employment

Imagination is essential – employers won't be queuing up to offer jobs.

• Contact employers and organise some visits to local workplaces. It is important to arrange this beforehand with employers, explaining the aim of a possible visit.

• Set up a time-limited work experience placement.

• Start to consider how much support the person might need, and check that resources are available to provide appropriate support.

Work experience

A work experience placement can be used as an opportunity for people to find out more about a particular type of job. It can also be a way of getting to know the individual in a work situation. Sometimes it can be part of a person's route towards a suitable paid job.

Work experience is an unpaid period of time spent in an ordinary workplace, finding out about a particular job or jobs. It does not guarantee a paid job for the individual who completes a placement. However, an employer could be approached to provide a reference for the person, to support future paid job applications. Regular review of placements is crucial. A placement should have clear boundaries and a time limit. It should not go on and on and on!

Setting up a placement

• Contact local companies (large and small) for possible placements.

• Check that the placement will offer the individual the right opportunities.

• Explain the aim of the placement to the employer.

• Be clear about the level of responsibility expected of the individual, and check that they will be supported as appropriate by the care staff team.

• Check the individual is covered by insurance while on the employer's premises.

• Check that the placement is a safe place to work. ALL employers have an obligation to abide by the Health and Safety at Work (etc) Act 1974.

• Find out whether an employer would be willing to meet any extra expenses such as fares and meals.

Sources of help: A set of two packs called *Work Experience on Employers' Premises* is available. The two packs, one aimed at care staff and one to use with people with learning disabilities, contain checklists, practical advice about setting up a placement, and other useful information.[1]

Looking for a job

There are several places where people look for jobs,these include job centres, newspapers, journals and staff vacancy boards. Use **all** the local available resources, and check whether there are any specialist agencies.

As part of the Employment Service for **all** job seekers, Placement, Assessment and Counselling Teams (PACTs) offer a comprehensive local service specifically for people with disabilities. Ask at your local Job Centre for information about the following:

DISABILITY EMPLOYMENT ADVISERS(DEAs))

Their work includes helping people with disabilities to find work which suits their skills. Sometimes the DEA may refer job seekers to local specialist training or assessment centres. DEAs cannot support people in the workplace, and therefore only place people who are ready to work independently. The DEA will also know more about the schemes mentioned below.

AIDS AND ADAPTATIONS

A free loan service to registered disabled people of certain aids and tools, to help them to gain or keep employment.

TRAVEL TO WORK GRANTS

Available to registered disabled people who are unable (due to their disability) to travel to work by public transport.

JOB INTRODUCTION SCHEME

Offers a financial incentive to employers for up to thirteen weeks to take on a disabled worker. This gives the new disabled worker an opportunity to learn the job and demonstrate their own capabilities to the employer.

SHELTERED PLACEMENT SCHEME

A wage subsidy scheme aimed specifically to support people who have more severe disabilities who wish to work in ordinary workplaces. Check with the DEA whether a scheme operates in your area.

JOB CLUB offers job seekers a place to seek vacancies (using the telephone, stationery and postage stamps) and a chance to meet other job seekers.

To gain access to some of the above services it is necessary to be a Registered Disabled Person (with the Employment Service) but it is not compulsory to register.

People with learning disabilities may need support to find their way round what is available. DEAs should have useful contacts with local employers, and information on current vacancies. You can agree beforehand that any support in the workplace would be provided by the care staff team.

Support in keeping a job

If a job search proves successful, it is important that support from the staff team continues. Support must be available in the workplace: on the job training is the best way of finding out how the person is getting on in their new role as a worker, and employers need to know that the job will be completed to the usual standard. So the staff member should work *alongside* the person with learning disabilities, until they are established. Don't forget people need to learn the routines and procedures related to the job, as well as the job itself.

The benefits maze

People looking for jobs will want to know how much extra they will have to spend as they wish if they are working. Care staff should support them to make informed choices based on the effect of earnings and other income on benefits.

Nearly every year there are changes in the rules and names of benefits. The following information can only give you a general idea of the way a person's benefits are calculated. It applies to adults (aged 18-60) with learning disabilities, and is intended to help you and those you work with to ask the right questions and check what you are told.

Many benefits are paid by the Benefits Agency (BA) on behalf of the Department of Social Security (DSS). All letters from the BA and copies of everything sent to them, must be kept safely. The person should also keep a diary of dates worked and earnings received, and a record of National Insurance contributions paid.

People can check how their own benefits are calculated by asking the BA for form A124 *How Your Income Support Is Worked Out*. People in registered residential care and nursing homes should ask for form A124BL.

Hostels, registered residential care homes and sheltered housing have different benefit rules. If you are not sure, ask your manager which type of residential care is being provided where you work.

From April 1993 local authorities will be involved in the administration of benefits for people in residential care.

Benefits for people with disabilities can be divided into three categories:
• money to help with the extra costs of disability
• benefits for people whose disability has affected their ability to work
• money to cover basic living costs such as housing and food.

Benefits to help with the extra costs of disability
• **Disability Living Allowance** (DLA) has a mobility component and a care component. People who used to get Mobility and/or Attendance Allowance get the equivalent DLA allowances. In April 1992 more people became eligible as lower levels of dependence were included.

DLA Mobility payments are not affected by earnings, neither do they reduce other benefit payments. DLA care payments are deducted from the income support paid to people living in registered residential care.

Benefits for people who have a disability which affects their ability to work
• **Severe Disablement Allowance** (SDA) is topped up by Income Support and/or Housing Benefit to meet basic needs.

• **Disability Premium** is added to the income support paid to people with long term disabilities.

People living in registered residential care are not eligible for the Disability Premium, but they have an "underlying entitlement" to the Disability Premium if they have proved to the BA that they have a disability which affects their ability to work. The best option for them if they want a job is to apply to have their paid part time work accepted as "therapeutic" earnings (see next page).

• **Disability Working Allowance** (DWA). This benefit tops up earnings of people with disabilities who are earning too much to continue receiving SDA. They must be working for at least 16 hours a week, and earning less than £90. The amount DWA adds to income is reduced as earnings increase, so that earnings of £90 a week get no DWA top-up at all. A person receiving DWA would also be eligible for

DLA benefits, Housing Benefit and other allowances for people on low pay.

It is unlikely to enable anyone to increase their income substantially. Its main advantage is that it enables a person with net pay between the therapeutic earnings limit and £90 to be recognised as being at a disadvantage in getting and keeping a job. They should be able to return to their previous benefits if they stop working within two years, as long as they can still prove that they have a significant disability.

Supported employment services have successfully challenged the notion that people with learning disabilities are incapable of work, but the benefits rules have not caught up with this. The rules make it difficult for a person dependent on support services at home and at work to gain much financially.

It is important to be honest about the amount of support a person needs to learn and keep a job so that they are not arbitrarily deprived of benefits, and also to be honest with the person with learning disabilities who may be expecting a significant rise in their standard of living.

Benefits to cover basic living expenses

• Income Support and Housing Benefit
People usually depend on these benefits for all housing, support, meals and personal spending money which are not covered by other income or benefits.

If you work in a registered residential care home you may be surprised how high the charges are. Most of the cost is to cover buying, maintaining, heating, staffing and furnishing the residential home, even if it is a small staffed house. Sometimes meals are included in the charge, other homes arrange for people to pay for food separately.

The "pocket money" allowance is small and has to cover clothes, entertainment, holidays, toiletries, and other personal costs such as cigarettes, magazines and stamps. Earning even a small amount can therefore make a difference to the choices available to a person with learning disabilities.

Benefits protection

There are three ways in which a person can earn money but still have some protection for their benefits within DSS regulations: Earnings Disregard, Therapeutic Earnings, or Trust Funds.

Earnings Disregard
The first fifteen pounds of earnings should not be deducted from the income support paid to a person who has a disability. It is not true that people with learning disabilities are not allowed to earn more than £15. However, any pay above this will be deducted pound for pound from Income Support, so that the working person with learning disabilities will have to start paying more of their personal "pocket money" costs from their earnings. This particularly affects people who depend on high Income Support to pay the fees for residential care homes.

Therapeutic Earnings
If the BA believes that a person with learning disabilities could earn enough to live on, they may lose their eligibility for SDA and would then be treated the same as any other unemployed person.

It is often helpful to begin with "therapeutic" earnings. This means that the BA accepts that the person is working part time as part of a training or rehabilitation scheme, and will continue to treat them as incapable of work. "Therapeutic earnings" are still affected by the £15 earnings disregard for Income Support. The BA will accept that work is "therapeutic" if:

a) the earnings are no more than the

SAMPLE LETTER TO A DOCTOR
asking for support to claim Therapeutic Earnings status

Dear Dr Clark

I am writing on behalf of one of your patients, Ms Carol Simpson, to ask for your help.

We have arranged for Ms Simpson to spend up to eight hours a week in supported employment, using social and work skills. This will include four hours office cleaning, such as hoovering, dusting, emptying waste bins and sweeping and washing floors. She will also be spending four hours in a sheltered workshop learning picture framing.

As she will be providing useful services during these sessions, she will receive allowances averaging £25 a week in total.

This work will differ from normal employment because Ms Simpson will be working under the constant supervision of instructors employed by a supported employment service for adults with learning disabilities. The instructors will provide Carol with on-the-job training and assessments.

Ms Simpson knows that her benefits will be reduced because she is earning. The first fifteen pounds should be disregarded. The remaining ten pounds will be deducted from her Income Support.

She will be entitled to continue to be treated as incapable of work, and to receive Severe Disablement Allowance if the Benefits Agency accepts that the work is of therapeutic value.

To qualify for this concession Ms Simpson needs a letter from you saying that as her doctor you agree that she can do these tasks and will benefit from this.

If you think there are any medical reasons for Ms Simpson to avoid certain types of work, we will take this into account in planning her activities.

If you need further information, please contact me on the above number.

Yours sincerely...

"therapeutic earnings limit" (£41.50 in 1992-3);

b) a doctor agrees that the person can do the work;

c) a doctor agrees that the work is "therapeutic" (if the work is organised and supported by a professional service such as a day centre, community team or supported employment service and will include on-the-job training and assessment this will help to establish its therapeutic value);

d) the BA is told about this **before** the person starts work. They should have written agreement from the BA, so allow several weeks for this process.

Above and overleaf are two sample letters which can be adapted to suit individual needs. Ms Carol Simpson is planning to work part time with the support of service workers.

The BA should be willing to continue to treat Carol as incapable of work as long as she only works according to the limits described in the letters.

If the BA believes that Carol is apparently capable of working longer hours under less special conditions she may be told that she is capable of work and should rely more on earnings rather than benefits. She would have the right to appeal against this decision.

SAMPLE LETTER TO LOCAL OFFICE OF THE BENEFITS AGENCY
asking for Therapeutic Earnings rule to be applied

Dear Sir or Madam,

RE: Ms Carol Simpson
Address and NATIONAL INSURANCE NUMBER (as shown on benefit book)

Ms Simpson is dependent on benefits as she has severe learning disabilities and a hearing impairment. She has no other income at present.

We have arranged for Ms Simpson to spend up to eight hours a week in supported employment, using social and work skills. This will include four hours office cleaning, such as hoovering, dusting, emptying waste bins and sweeping and washing floors, and also four hours in a sheltered workshop learning picture framing.

As she will be providing useful services during these sessions, she will receive allowances averaging £25 a week in total.

This work will be different from normal employment because Ms Simpson will be working under the constant supervision of instructors employed by a supported employment service for adults with learning disabilities. The instructors will provide Carol with on-the-job training and assessments.

Ms Simpson expects that her Income Support will be reduced by ten pounds once she starts earning, calculated according to the following rules:

a) Fifteen pounds should be disregarded as Ms Simpson has disabilities which affect her ability to earn a living.

b) The tasks involved have therapeutic value (the therapeutic earnings rule for people on Invalidity Benefit or Severe Disablement Allowance).

c) Her doctor agrees that she can do these tasks and will benefit from this project (see enclosed letter).

d) Her total earnings are below the Therapeutic Earnings Limit
Ms Simpson would like to begin her work as soon as possible.

Please confirm within two weeks that Ms Simpson's benefits will not be reduced by more than ten pounds and that she will continue to be treated as incapable of work under the therapeutic earnings rule.

Yours faithfully...

Trust Funds

Regular cash payments from a trust are usually treated as unearned income. An equivalent amount is deducted from income support so that a person gains nothing unless they earn enough not to need income support at all.

Some employment schemes have arranged for a trust to receive regular payments from someone's earnings. They can then apply to the trust for occasional non-essential "gifts" such as a holiday or audio equipment. This should not affect benefits. You must check the current rules very carefully before recommending this.

Other income

If a person has another source of regular unearned income such as National Insurance benefits, compensation, transition payments, rent from property or interest from savings, they need independent advice from a welfare rights adviser or law centre before they start work, as there are complicated rules and legal judgements which will affect them. This also applies to people with learning disabilities who are living with a partner or who have dependents.

Other costs

It is important to recognise any extra costs involved in work, including refreshments, fares, clothing and equipment. People need to find out what help is available from various sources, including the BA. Free meals at work do not affect a person's benefits, but if an employer pays fares to work this will be treated as income.

Sources of help

To make effective use of the following sources of help, a person needs to have a list of their current benefits, savings and other income, and to know what type of residential service they are using.

Citizen's Advice Bureaux

These give confidential advice on many subjects. Most towns have self-help groups for people with disabilities which give advice and support and lobby for improvements in benefits and services.

Disability Rights Handbook

This is published every year, with supplements to keep it up to date. Produced by The Disability Alliance Educational and Research Association, Universal House, 88-94 Wentworth Street, London E1 7SA. Tel: 071 247 8776.

DSS Freeline for people with disabilities. Tel: 0800 882200.

This is a free telephone service. The advice workers do not have access to individual files, but they will answer general questions and send you leaflets.

Points to remember

Finding and keeping a job

1. Work out what support the individual needs to learn the job.
2. Ensure that support is consistent and is focused on the individual learning the job (use skills teaching techniques; keep records of progress made).
3. Provide the right help with routines and procedures e.g. reporting sickness, clocking in on time, maintaining a uniform.
4. Be available for the employer, in case they have any problems. If the job responsibilities change, a period of re training may be required.
5. It is better to succeed than to be over-ambitious. If the choice is between supporting someone consistently in part time work, or a full time job in which they will be left to cope on their own because of the competing demands on your time, go for the part time option.

Benefits

1. Know what benefits the individual should be receiving.
2. Know the effect of earnings on these benefits.
3. Support an individual to get independent advice if necessary.
4. Help them make informed choices.
5. Help them get as many other gains from working as possible, as well as money.
6. Make sure the individual is getting whatever help is available with costs related to work, such as fares, meals and clothing.

Resources

1. *Work Experience on Employers' Premises*. Two packs available from Futures to Work For, c/o Connect, PO Box 30, Avon House North, St. James Barton, Bristol BS99 7NB. Tel: 0272 290777. Cost £8.00 (incl. P&P.) The pack is available free to services within the County of Avon.

CHAPTER 12

Leisure and recreation

John Brennan

• Which activity? An individual choice • Integration wherever possible: using leisure centres, local clubs and societies • Steps towards independence

Most people confuse "leisure" with spare time, but spare time in itself can soon lead to boredom if you do not put some thought and planning into how you spend it.

You may spend some of the time doing nothing or very little, or it you may put all your time and vast amounts of energy and expense into a leisure activity. Most people settle for something in the middle of these two extremes.

Integration

Leisure is now big business and those who run leisure activities are sure to be interested in increasing the number of people using their centres.

Most of the things that go on in special clubs or classes for people with learning disabilities are also going on somewhere in a more normal setting. Also, with help from the media, the public have become a little more enlightened about the needs and rights of the people we work with. We can help further by enabling them to use normal leisure and recreational facilities even if it means adjusting and adapting the activity to accommodate them. Involving people with a learning disability in ordinary leisure pursuits in the local area can be a good way of educating the public to adjust to and accept them. It also opens opportunities for the person with a learning disability to be befriended, or make friends in their own right.

Trying things out

Leisure pursuits are a matter of personal choice, which people can take up or leave at will. Most of us tend to try out a number of recreation and leisure activities. If we look under our stairs or on top of our wardrobe we are likely to find reminders and leftovers of many activities we were involved with in the past.

People with learning disabilities should also be helped acquire items on top of their wardrobes. But because they need help in many areas of everyday living, they will need help and guidance on using the ordinary leisure and recreational activities in the areas in which they live.

Exploring your area

Your first step should be an assessment of the leisure opportunities available locally. The local library is a good place to begin; they usually carry a list of all clubs and societies in the area, and they will provide you with the names and addresses of their secretaries. The names of societies will give you lots of new ideas for activities you would not otherwise have thought of.

Choosing an activity

Some people will need help and guidance in selecting a leisure activity. Sometimes it helps if the helper or member of care staff suggests an activity which they like themselves; this can be a big step towards shared success. Care staff should of course be aware that some activities carry an element of risk, and this should be assessed and discussed.

Funding for a new activity may also have to be thought about, as there may be expenses for equipment and/or staff support, travel etc. It can be more economical if an activity begins with staff support, and at a later date this support is transferred to a volunteer or befriender. Involving the person in an activity out of the house can put extra demands on the staff team and the rota, so it will need the full co-operation of the other members of staff. In some cases it will appear that job descriptions do not fit in with some of the leisure activities envisaged. Staff rotas and working hours have to be flexible enough to cope with weekends and other times when normal leisure activities happen. So as you can see it will in many cases mean a team effort to make things happen and keep them happening.

The best way for anyone to choose an activity is to try it out a few times, with staff involved and observing carefully what interest is shown. Television programmes, photographs, pictures cut from magazines can also help when trying to discuss with someone what they might be interested in. When a choice is made, a more detailed assessment of the activity should follow.

Planning

When the chosen activity has been agreed by everyone involved, further preparatory work and research will begin. Say in this case walking has been chosen, the first

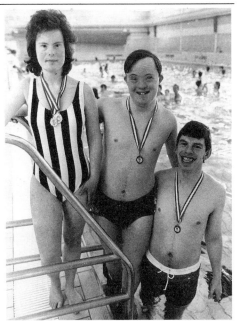

Photo: Mencap

What starts as a leisure activity could open the door to many new challenges. The sky's the limit!

questions to consider are:

- Where will this walking take place?
- How long should it be?
- What will be needed?
- Will it lead on to anything interesting? Joining a Rambling Club maybe?

Where will the walk take place?

With information from your local library or local authority you can locate a local walk as near as possible to where the person lives. Many of these walks may be within local country parks with well laid out marked routes. They are usually marked out in various lengths, from short to long. It is advisable to try this walk to assess any unforeseen problems:

- How many gates and stiles are there? Will they be difficult for the person to manage?
- Are there any animals which may cause a problem, such as a dog dashing out barking? You will be able to use your background knowledge of the person to anticipate any problems.

How long should the walk be?

Your knowledge of the individual and your own abilities should help you make a decision on the length of the walk (best to keep it short to begin with).

What is needed?

People should be suitably dressed for walking. You need:

1. Good shoes or boots.
2. Light, waterproof clothing.
3. Small haversack.
4. Something to eat and drink.
5. Some information on the walk (this can usually be acquired from the library or your local authority. Pictorial guides can be purchased for some town walks. These are very useful because they provide an opportunity for the person to participate in identifying places and things on the walks, leading eventually to a sense of achievement if someone becomes able to find their own way on the walk.

The next step

When the person has been walking a while and obviously enjoys the activity, they could graduate to longer and more difficult walks. The next step would be to contact a local rambling club. They usually advertise their local walks in the newspapers, giving the meeting place, length of walk and time. If not, the club can be contacted via the local library.

How is this step to be taken? Should a staff member just turn up at one of the advertised walks to assess what is involved in becoming a member of the club? Or should they contact the secretary and discuss the possibility of a person with a learning difficulty joining the rambling club?

Valued citizens do not usually telephone in advance to find out if they will be allowed to take part in club activities. This would suggest not doing so on behalf of a person with a learning disability. Visits to the club by care staff are useful however, to find out whether they have any vacancies for new members, and whether it is a suitable club to join.

It may be a good idea for you to go on one of the club walks as a taster, to assess the type of walk and the company. If all seems well, you can both try out a few of the club walks together before joining.

If all goes well, the person is now involved in a normal club activity in the community, with the opportunity to meet new people, to move away from the care staff and become more independent with the help of club members who may be able to offer support during the walks.

If all this is successful it is possible to move on with the club or in your own small party to hostelling or rambling holidays, so "the sky is the limit".

When the person has reached this stage of the activity, it will open the door to many more challenges, and possibly in a number of years someone will ask why are they keeping their old worn walking shoes on top of their wardrobe!

Free to choose

Choosing walking as just one example from the long list of possible activities, I have described how I introduced a small number of people who attended a local social education centre to this leisure activity. Their interest persisted, and they became quite knowledgeable about the activity, moving on to walking with local clubs, and to using hostels.

Whichever activity is chosen, careful planning and research, are essential to make it successful and enjoyable. It will only be pleasurable if the people with learning disabilities are free to choose whether and when to participate.

CHAPTER 13

Meeting the needs of Black people

Peter Ferns

• What is racism? What is race equality? • Some good and bad ways we can respond to racism • Challenging stereotypes • Building on the "hidden talents" and strengths of Black people • Valuing cultural diversity • Increasing self-esteem and confidence • Helping people speak for themselves and reclaim their rights

What is so different about Black people, you may ask, that they have a special chapter of this book devoted to them? There are no differences between Black and white people in their basic needs for shelter, food, warmth, or the care they need because of disability. But there *are* differences in life experiences and culture, which mean that some needs have to be met in different ways.

Because of racism in our society, Black people are an oppressed group who experience discrimination and disadvantage in their everyday lives. So in caring for them their experiences must be taken into account, and services must both challenge racism and work to stop racism happening.

"Black" is used as a political term to stand for solidarity or togetherness for people who experience racism because of their skin colour. By using the term "Black", it is hoped to give people support and confidence to stand up against racism and not feel isolated. It is spelled here with a capital letter to remind us that it is a political term and not just a reference to colour.

What is racism ?

Racism is a word to describe racial *prejudice*, that is negative attitudes and beliefs about Black people, and racial *discrimination*, which is unfair behaviour towards a group of people because of their skin colour. Thus it involves the abuse of power by white people, who have more power in a society which has been racist for a long time, and has taken power away from Black people in many different ways.

Racism can be experienced on two levels: between individuals, or from institutions and organisations in society such as education, housing authorities, the legal system, health and social services. There is a great deal of evidence that racism is still a big problem for Black people in Britain today.

What is race equality ?

Race equality involves changing white people's negative attitudes towards Black people, introducing ways of thinking about people which value their racial and cultural differences. A second aspect of race equality is to put into place equal opportunities policies and other measures to deal with institutional discrimination and safeguard Black people's rights to fair treatment by those organisations. The third aspect of race equality is to empower Black people, which means to support Black people in taking more control over their own lives and to work actively against racism in society.

Responding to racism

How do white people, and organisations run mainly by white people, respond to racism? The following are examples of unhelpful responses often made when racism and racist practices are challenged:

• **"It's not my concern."** This comes from a belief that racism is the concern of Black people, and is not really to do with white people's attitudes and behaviour. So, for instance, people mistakenly believe that racism can only happen if you have Black people present.

• **"Black people should fit into British culture."** This assumes that British culture is only white and European, not the mix of cultures it actually is. It is also another way of saying that white British culture is best and that white people have nothing to learn from other cultures.

• **"There's no racism here."** This comes from a reluctance to accept the unpleasant reality that Britain still has a racist society which treats Black people unfairly. Racism is bound to affect every organisation in this country because it is part of so many things in society.

• **"I treat everyone the same."** This is a colour-blind approach which does not accept the real life experiences of Black people who *are* treated differently. "The same" often means being treated as if you are white. Anyway, equality does not mean being treated the same, it means equal

respect for people's rights, experiences and their individual needs.

• **"Black people should have their own services."** This is a way of avoiding responsibility for changing mainstream services so that they are accessible and appropriate for Black people. Black-led services or Black groups are useful and important in a situation of inequality, but these services should not be the only option available for Black people. Race equality approaches should open more choices for Black people, not fewer.

• **"I need to know about Black people's cultures."** There is nothing wrong with wanting to know more about a person's culture but care must be taken not to stereotype and make assumptions about people based on their culture. It is very difficult to fully understand a person's culture. So the best thing to do is to treat the person and their family as experts and to respect the person's culture as an important aspect of their care.

Have you heard any of these responses in your services? What would you answer now if somebody said these things to you again?

Experiences of racism

Black people with learning disabilities experience racism in the following ways:

• Being racially stereotyped because of your skin colour as well as being stereotyped as a person with learning disability. A stereotype is where a person is assumed to have particular characteristics or behaviours because they belong to an identified group in society. So stereotypes are a barrier to seeing a person as an individual, and to appreciating their individual skills and talents.

• Not having your skills and abilities recognised partly because people around you do not understand your cultural skills and abilities.

• Being seen as negatively different because of your culture.

• Losing self confidence, self esteem, racial and cultural identity and being treated as if you were white.

• Not being listened to; having your wishes and preferences ignored.

• Having people who do not understand your culture decide what is best for you.

• Having your family and community ties weakened when these ties are essential for you to survive racism.

• Being unsure about your rights and how to stand up for them and make a complaint.

• Having to deal with organisations that do not uphold equal rights for Black people and disabled people.

• Having your views about service quality ignored.

Think of the Black people you have worked with or known about. Did they have similar experiences?

Working for Race Equality

Because care services are there to help people and enable them to gain more control over their own lives, services cannot help Black people effectively unless institutional racism is recognised and tackled. Black people are unlikely to use services if they can see them operating in a discriminatory way. The services offered must meet Black people's needs in a way that does not offend people and suits them in terms of traditions, customs or religious beliefs. If these kinds of changes in services do not happen, care services will continue to be effectively denied to many Black communities and remain inaccessible and inappropriate. In this way services will strengthen racism in society rather than making a valuable contribution to greater race equality.

Care workers must also take responsibility for their practice if services are to work for race equality. One committed care worker in an establishment can make a great deal of difference to the day to day experience of the individuals they work with. Each of the following topics ends up with some practical suggestions for positive things you can do:

Challenging stereotypes

Clear evidence of stereotyping can be found in written records. For instance, Asian parents may be described as too rigid and interfering in the lives of their adult daughter or son. The way information is recorded and gathered often has a big effect on the assessment of needs and the subsequent services provided. The needs of Black people and their families are often perceived through the eyes of white assessors who have little or no understanding of the family's culture, but have biased attitudes about Black people gained from a racist society.

Evidence of stereotyping can also be found in the way that services treat Black people but this evidence is more difficult to collect. For instance, African Caribbean young men are often perceived as being more "aggressive" and "threatening" by staff, a common stereotype projected by the newspapers and television programmes. This has led to Black young men being labelled more readily as having "challenging" behaviours and being placed in more restrictive living situations.

Things to do
• Look through written records and reports of Black people. Do they use racist language or put forward stereotyped views? You can point this out to managers.

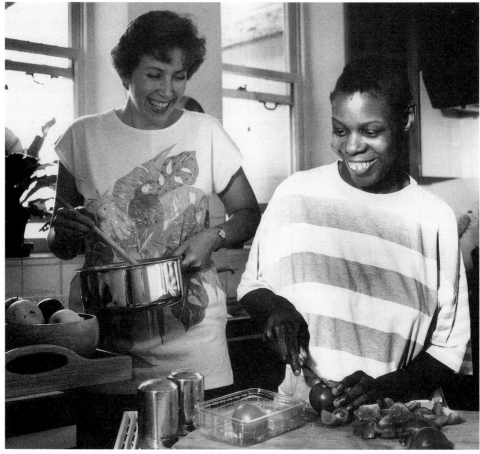

Photo: Debbie Humphry/Mencap

Offering everyone food from different cultures is a good way of valuing cultural diversity.

• Take a look at the way your service meets the needs of Black people. Are there any patterns, for example Black people being seen more readily as "problems", or in the way they are dealt with as a result?

• Is your service in an area where there are Black people, and is this mix of people reflected in your group? If you do have few or no Black people, why is this? What is putting them off?

Building on strengths

Black people often have "hidden talents" because their skills are not recognised in care settings that are culturally very different from the way of life they are accustomed to. For instance, they may be able to cook types of food that are never mentioned in the care setting, or make their own traditional clothes, which is a less common skill in modern British society. They may have complex language skills in their own language which are overlooked within the service, so they are quite literally silenced. They may also be knowledgeable about their own customs and religion; this often goes unrecognised by care establishments.

The behaviour of Black people is often seen as being problematic by care staff, when there has been no acknowledgement of the racism they are very likely to face. If Black people are described as displaying "inappropriate" or "anti-social" behaviour it has to be asked first whether they have been reacting to a racist care setting where their needs have been neither recognised nor met.

Viewing people's behaviour in this way may lead care staff to see it as an understandable way of asserting personal rights, even though the person may need help in finding appropriate ways of asserting their rights. The so-called "problem behaviour" may in fact be a strength, as it is an indication of their awareness of being Black, awareness of personal rights and their determination to reclaim those rights.

Valuing cultural diversity

The cultures of Black people are portrayed through negative images in many ways, and this makes it even more important for services to carry positive images of Britain as a multicultural society. Black people will feel more comfortable in surroundings that reflect their own cultures in some way such as posters, pictures, books. It is also important to respect people's culture in an active way. For instance, by celebrating different festivals or learning a little about people's different languages and customs.

Things to do
• Find out about some major festivals from Black cultures. When do they happen and why do people celebrate these festivals?
• Get some books and posters that give a positive view of a Black culture.
• Find out about the different games that are played in Black cultures.

Increasing self-esteem

Increasing self-confidence, self-esteem, racial and cultural identity – this issue is particularly important for people whose self-esteem has been threatened through racism. Racial and cultural identity are important for Black people to grow, develop and maintain a healthy personality, where they feel happy to be Black and to have a different culture from white people around them when and if they wish.

Hair and skin care
An essential part of personal identity is personal appearance, and for Black people it is important to pay attention to the cultural factors that come into dress, hair and skin care and personal hygiene.

For instance, it is very important for African Caribbean people to have regular combing of their hair with the use of the appropriate hair gels and fashionable hair styles. Failure to do this will result in matted hair in a short period of time, which can quickly necessitate cutting a person's hair in order to comb it properly. Sikhs do not usually have their hair cut but require hair styling to a "top-knot" and the application of special oils.

Skin care for African Caribbean people has also been conspicuously neglected in care establishments, resulting in dry, flaking skin due to the lack of appropriate skin oils. Information about hair and skin care is available through various publications (see Resource list). Care establishments could make links with local hairdressers and beauticians who specialise in Black hair and skin care.

Food is another aspect of basic care where cultural and religious needs are ignored or inadequately catered for. It is a basic right to have food that is your own choice, but sadly in many care establishments such choice is denied to both Black and white people. The impact on Black people can be worse, because the food offered is neither acceptable to their religion nor culturally familiar. Offering everyone foods from different cultures can be a good way of valuing cultural diversity.

Tradition and history

Where Black people have been in institutional care for a long period of time and have had little or no contact with Black communities or their families, it is likely that they may not have a strong racial or cultural identity and may even have negative feelings towards other Black people. In this situation it is vitally important for care workers to help them gain a positive view of their own racial identity and cultural heritage. Black people should be offered opportunities to learn more about their family's culture, traditions and history of their community. If a Black person does not have English as their first language, it would be necessary for care workers to enable them to communicate in their first language with another person from their community. Workers could even learn a few common words of that person's language and speak to them directly in a small way.

Things to do

• Find out where the local Black people go to have their hair done and where they buy oils and lotions for skin and hair care.
• Find out how to cook a recipe from a Black culture and where you would buy the ingredients.

Speaking for themselves

One of the first things that is needed for a person to speak for themselves is the kind of self-confidence and strong personal identity discussed above. Another important factor is communication skills, and Black people may have the additional barrier of not having English as their first language. Workers should provide opportunities for Black people to speak for themselves. Holding residents' meetings and encouraging people to take responsibility in conducting and controlling meetings, are good ways of

practising communication skills.

Self advocacy groups are an excellent way of both practising communication skills and empowering users to speak for themselves. Black self advocacy groups are particularly useful for Black people to discuss issues about coping with racism and for Black empowerment where Black people are helped in the group to feel confident and positive about Black.

Things to do

• Find out if there are any self advocacy groups in your area. If there are none, how could you help to get one started?

• Try to start having regular meetings for people with learning disabilities if you don't have them at present. If you do have meetings, do people with learning disabilities really have control over them?

• Look into the possibility of starting a group for Black people with learning disabilities, or enabling people to join a Black group in the community.

Making decisions

People who are not used to being asked about their opinions soon lose the skills to communicate their choices, and may even be afraid of choosing. Care workers have to support people in identifying their preferences and making choices.

Knowing your options and making choices also requires power and influence in decisions to bring choices into effect. Care organisations have to be made more sensitive to the views of people with learning disabilities, giving them more say in the way services assist them and especially in the major decisions that affect their lives.

Increased sensitivity in the organisation starts with listening more carefully to what people with learning disabilities are saying, and care staff, because they have most contact, are in a good position to listen and stand up for their views. Workers can also make sure that people with learning disabilities and their families are more aware of their rights and have accurate information about services so that people can speak up for themselves from a position of knowledge.

The language staff use must be clear, understandable and free from jargon. If people and their families do not have English as their first language, then the use of interpreters should be considered.

Things to do
• Make sure Black people and their families have enough information about your service, in their first language if necessary.
• Check that Black people and their families are fully involved in all the important decisions made about them. If not, find out what the barriers are and try to remove them.

Family and community

For Black people, the support and strength gained from family and community is very important in surviving racism in everyday life. Black disabled people are more at risk of feeling isolated because Black communities themselves may well need help in understanding and meeting the needs of disabled people. So maintaining social links in their preferred culture is vital for the growth and development of Black people with learning disabilities.

The most important link here is often the Black person's family. Care workers should make great efforts to contact families and encourage links. Giving regular information about the individual's wellbeing and progress builds up channels of communication. Enabling families to be actively involved in care can build trust, restore the family's confidence and counteract any feelings of guilt they may have had. Many Black families work together on the basis of strong family duty, and a sense of failure in that duty can bring much pain and guilt. A partnership between care workers and Black families should be offered to families, and may well be welcomed.

Care workers should also be aware of any local Black resources that could be of interest. Places such as Black community centres, religious establishments and clubs, can be valuable resources in helping people make new relationships with ordinary members of the Black community. Black organisations may require help and advice in welcoming Black disabled people, and care organisations can provide information and advice about disability to improve access for Black disabled people.

Things to do
• Actively involve a Black family in the individual's care, even if it is only in a small way.
• Find ways of improving the channels of communication between the care establishment and Black families, for example by having a special meeting for Black families. Make sure regular information about the individual is given to their family.
• Find out about local Black groups and have this information available.

Rights and complaints

If someone has difficulty in speaking for themselves, it is important to try and get an independent person to represent their interests (and no one else's). An independent "advocate" can be a friend, a volunteer such as a Citizen Advocate or some kind of paid advocate from an independent organisation. It is possible to use a family member in some instances but care has to be taken that the family member does not represent their own interests rather than the individual's. For Black people it would be best to have a Black advocate and for people who speak little or no English an advocate who can translate would be ideal.

Care workers should make themselves familiar with their organisation's complaints procedure so that they can give accurate information about the procedure to users and their families. It would be useful to keep leaflets about the complaints procedure available at your workplace, and have translated leaflets if necessary.

Things to do

• See if there are any local advocacy schemes in your area. Raise the issue of getting independent advocates (particularly for people who cannot speak for themselves) with the staff team.

• Find out what your organisation's complaints procedure is and get some suitable information or leaflets to pass on to Black people and their families.

Equal opportunities

It seems obvious to tell you to read your organisation's Equal Opportunities Policy, but it is surprising the number of people who are not even sure what such policies say. Read the policy then ask questions of your manager if you are unsure about anything.

If you are working for a good organisation, there may also be a Race Equality Strategy, which is a set of plans to put the policy into operation, and practice guidelines which give workers practical ways of using the policy in the workplace. It is the responsibility of every employee of the organisation to put the policy into practice, and workers will have to think about the type of training they need to

bring race equality into their practice. If care staff are unsure about working with Black people, some of the more progressive organisations may have Race Advisers to support and advise staff in practical, "on-the-job" strategies. It may be best to start the whole process of improving practice with a statement of the team's commitment to develop race equality, so that individual workers will feel supported in their efforts to improve their personal practice.

Things to do

• Make sure that you are familiar with and understand your organisation's Equal Opportunities Policy.

• Ask your team and your manager how you are implementing this policy in your establishment.

• Think about your own training needs in the area of race equality, and how you can get these training needs met.

Quality assurance

It is easier to involve people in monitoring quality of services if there is a system for examining the service you give. Such systems are often called Quality Assurance systems: people with learning disabilities and their families should have a central role, and any judgements made must be based on their views.

An effective way to monitor the service you are giving is to ask people about their experience of your service, record their views at regular intervals – individually or in groups – and report back to managers. Black people may need help to participate in such groups, and you should watch that staff do not make it difficult for people to say what they really think. See Chapter 4 on Individual Planning.

Resources

"Being Black with Learning Difficulties" by

Experiences of Racism	**Working for Equality**
1. Being racially stereotyped.	1. Challenging stereotypes of Black people.
2. Not having your skills and abilities recognised.	2. Recognising and building on the strengths of Black users.
3. Being seen as negatively different because of your culture.	3. Valuing cultural diversity.
4. Losing self-confidence, racial and cultural identity.	4. Increasing self-confidence, racial and cultural identity.
5. Not being listened to.	5. Enabling people to speak for themselves.
6. Having people who do not understand your culture decide what's best for you.	6. Increasing users' influence in decision-making.
7. Having your family and community ties weakened.	7. Strengthening family and community networks of Black people.
8. Being unsure about your rights and how to make a complaint.	8. Making sure that Black people understand their rights and know how to make a complaint.
9. Having to deal with organisations which do not uphold equal rights for Black people or disabled people.	9. Supporting and carrying out Equal Opportunities Policies.
10. Having your views about service quality ignored.	10. Involving people with learning disabilities in monitoring the quality of services.

POINTS TO REMEMBER: On the left are common experiences of racism; on the right are positive changes you can work for in each case.

a Black Advocacy Group and Peter Ferns. In *Changing the Balance - power and people who use services.* published by NCVO - Community Care Project, 1991.
Afro skin, hair care and recipes - booklet from the Commission for Racial Equality, and

Hair Care by Carol Baxter, National Extension College for Training in Health and Race. Also available from CRE.
Black Beauty and Hair magazine, Hawker Publications, 13 Park House, 140 Battersea Park Road, London SW11 4NB.

CHAPTER 14

Mealtimes and personal care

Barbara Ogden and Pauline Gee

• *Expressing our respect for people through good physical care* • *Mealtimes, choice, help with feeding* • *Help and support in personal care* • *Incontinence*

This chapter looks at how we can offer the best physical care to those people with learning disabilities who rely on care staff for help with eating, bathing and toileting. These issues are sometimes shunted into the background, and thought of as a bit of a chore, the unglamorous side of our job. The reality is that for those people who need help, the standard of care we achieve in these areas is central to people's wellbeing. It is no good us talking about *quality, rights, dignity* or using any other popular "buzz" words, unless we can put these commitments into practice in the way we assist people with learning disabilities to meet their basic everyday needs.

Eating and drinking

Meal times for most of us are a social occasion, relaxed and enjoyable. This should be our aim for the people we support.

To ensure that people are relaxed and able to enjoy their meal, you can make sure they have the opportunity to go to the toilet beforehand, that their clothes are dry and comfortable, that they are sitting in an upright position and the table is at a height where they can reach and see

their food. Unless it is absolutely necessary people should not separated from others when eating their meals.

Presentation and choice

The menu for meals should not be rigid. Many people with learning disabilities now contribute to choosing food and planning menus, either by meeting as a group and discussing the menu on a weekly or monthly basis, or by individuals choosing meals in turn. However this is achieved, it is important that they have a major part in the choice and preparation of meals. For people who have a severe learning disability, this can be achieved by care staff noting their likes and dislikes and communicating with the rest of the care team. People from ethnic minorities should be offered food which is in keeping with their preferences and religious beliefs.

Times of the meals should not be rigid. As far as possible they should suit the majority, but also allow for flexibility taking into account people's lifestyles and various activities.

It is also important to bear in mind people's varying dietary needs, their age, and their ability to chew and digest food.

Someone with dentures may find it difficult to chew tough food, such as steak. All food should be made as palatable as possible, and how it looks on the plate is important, so make sure food is cut up carefully; or if a soft or liquidised diet is needed, see that all parts of the meal are liquidised individually. Not only will this be more pleasing to the eye, but care staff will be able to identify any parts of the meal which the person dislikes.

Aids and equipment

To enable people to be as independent as possible, there are a variety of different aids and equipment available, such as plate guards, non-slip mats, adapted cutlery. An occupational therapist will be able to give you advice or information on this. Aids can also be obtained from the Disabled Living Foundation or Keep Able centres, or many large branches of Boots. It is important to find the best method of supporting someone who has additional physical disabilities, so advice should be sought from a speech and language therapist on swallowing and chewing, and a physiotherapist could give advice on seating.

If you need to physically help someone to eat, this should always be done on a one to one basis, and the person must be given enough time to chew and digest the food. The next mouthful should always be offered at a pace that suits that individual. This can be done by encouraging the person to indicate when they are ready for the next mouthful, either verbally, by gesture or by eye pointing.

Small amounts of food should be offered at a time and the person should also have the opportunity to drink during the meal. This is particularly important if someone has swallowing difficulties, and it is vital to ensure that food and fluids are not breathed into the lungs; this could lead to pneumonia or even sudden death from choking.

Food should be at a comfortable, palatable temperature. It should not be allowed to become cold (likely if person is a slow eater). You must also ensure food is not too hot, especially if it has been heated in a microwave oven.

Nutrition

Everyone should be encouraged to eat a well balanced diet. They should be enabled to make an informed choice about their preferences, including for example to be a vegetarian if they want to, and about what makes up a healthy balanced diet.

A balanced diet involves choosing from all the food groups, to make sure you get the protein, fat, carbohydrate, minerals and vitamins you need. Here are some common food sources of the important nutrients:

> **Protein** for growth and healing – in meat, fish, eggs, milk, cheese, yoghurt, nuts, beans and lentils, bread.
>
> **Carbohydrate** for energy – in bread, flour, pasta, rice, cereals, sugar, fruit and vegetables.
>
> **Fats** – in meat, fish, chicken, milk, cream, butter, oils, biscuits and cakes.
>
> **Fibre** to prevent constipation and bowel disorders – in fruit, vegetables, wholegrain and oat cereals and baking, wholemeal bread, beans and lentils.
>
> **Calcium** for strong bones and teeth – in milk, cheese and yoghurt, canned fish, green leafy vegetables, white bread.
>
> **Vitamin C** - potatoes, citrus fruit such as oranges, fruit juice, green vegetables, berry fruits.

If individuals are receiving special diets such as PKU (Phenylketonuria), gluten free, diabetic, reduced fat, low salt, low cholesterol, then advice can be sought from a dietician or GP. All staff should be told about the diet and given consistent guidelines about what the person can eat at home or at a restaurant or take-away.

Helping with bathing

The room should be warm. All toiletries, towels, flannels, whatever you need should be in the bathroom ready for use, to avoid having to leave the bathroom to fetch anything, and make sure the person won't be moved about half-dressed. The water temperature should be comfortable and kept as warm as the person likes it. People should be helped to choose their own toiletries, and there should be in the bathroom a choice of clothes or dressing gown and slippers.

Bathing aids

For people with added disabilities there is a range of equipment and adaptations available. Advice should be sought from an occupational therapist. If the person needs help with transferring, a physiotherapist should advise you on the best method. Both bath hoists and commodes are useful pieces of equipment, but commodes should never be used to wheel someone from room to room: this is undignified and degrading.

Taking risks

If someone does not wish to have a member of staff in the bathroom with them, this choice should be respected wherever possible. It may be necessary to assess the level of support the person needs and weigh up the amount of risk involved. It may be possible to take steps to reduce risk, as in the example above

Gemma was 25 years old, and lived in a staffed house. She had a mild learning disability and severe epilepsy which was poorly controlled.

Gemma did not want a member of staff sitting in the bathroom with her. Staff discussed with Gemma what could happen if she had a seizure in the bath.

What would you do in this situation?

1. Ignore Gemma's wishes, and sit in the bathroom.

2. Discuss with the consultant or GP ways of controlling Gemma's seizures better.

3. Meet with Gemma and the staff team to identify the risks.

In the end it was decided that a member of staff should stay with Gemma, but that the service would buy and use shower screens round the bath. That way the need for privacy could be met safely.

Another important aspect of personal care is care of the mouth and teeth. This is covered in Chapter 17 on health care.

Helping with continence

Think about how you can help people stay continent and respect their personal dignity at the same time. You can ask people discreetly in good time if they wish to use the toilet. You can make sure toilet doors are shut to preserve privacy. You can monitor how often an individual needs to use the toilet and plan a timetable accordingly. You may feel it is helpful to congratulate someone on successful use of the toilet, but do be sensitive – don't broadcast across the house what they have produced!

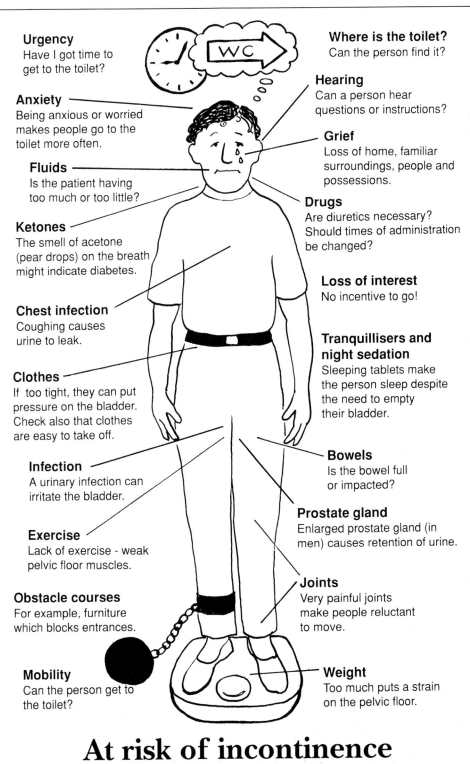

Urgency
Have I got time to
get to the toilet?

Anxiety
Being anxious or worried
makes people go to the
toilet more often.

Fluids
Is the patient having
too much or too little?

Ketones
The smell of acetone
(pear drops) on the breath
might indicate diabetes.

Chest infection
Coughing causes
urine to leak.

Clothes
If too tight, they can put
pressure on the bladder.
Check also that clothes
are easy to take off.

Infection
A urinary infection can
irritate the bladder.

Exercise
Lack of exercise - weak
pelvic floor muscles.

Obstacle courses
For example, furniture
which blocks entrances.

Mobility
Can the person get to
the toilet?

Where is the toilet?
Can the person find it?

Hearing
Can a person hear
questions or instructions?

Grief
Loss of home, familiar
surroundings, people and
possessions.

Drugs
Are diuretics necessary?
Should times of administration
be changed?

Loss of interest
No incentive to go!

**Tranquillisers and
night sedation**
Sleeping tablets make
the person sleep despite
the need to empty
their bladder.

Bowels
Is the bowel full
or impacted?

Prostate gland
Enlarged prostate gland (in
men) causes retention of urine.

Joints
Very painful joints
make people reluctant
to move.

Weight
Too much puts a strain
on the pelvic floor.

Eve Morris

At risk of incontinence

Incontinence

There are many possible reasons for incontinence (see the chart on page 113). You should be particularly concerned if someone who is normally continent suddenly becomes incontinent. Medical advice should be sought, as it could indicate a bladder infection or other medical problem, or sometimes even a psychological trauma or stress.

There are several different kinds of incontinence:

Stress incontinence
This is when the bladder leaks during coughing, sneezing, laughing, lifting, bending, jogging or running, or any sudden physical exercise. Confusingly perhaps, the term does not mean the mental stress that people experience perhaps at work or if they have personal problems, but the physical stress which is suddenly put on the muscles.

Urge incontinence
This is where people get a strong urge to go to the toilet with no advance warning. Sometimes the urge is so strong they are unable to reach the toilet quickly enough.

Dribble incontinence flow
This type of incontinence may occur because the bladder does not empty properly. This means that as the body drains more urine into the already full bladder, some leakage occurs.

Nocturnal enuresis (bed wetting)
This occurs when someone has not gained control over their bladder at night.

There are many aids available to maintain continence: for example pads, special pants, catheters, bottles. However some people are unable to maintain continence independently and need help and support from staff. Advice should be sought from either a Continence Adviser, Community Nurse for People with Learning Disabilities, or District Nurse.

Observe what happens and consult your GP or a nurse, who will help you work out the underlying cause of the person's incontinence, and draw up an appropriate care regime. Restricting the amount of fluid the person drinks is not helpful (unless they drink really excessive amounts) and might encourage bladder infection.

Sometimes people do not know they have wet themselves, and staff should tackle this with tact and sensitivity. People should not be left in wet clothes or treated in a way which makes them feel punished or humiliated. However irritating it is to have to keep changing someone, it is unlikely that it is being done deliberately. You will need to work out a system, as a staff group, which enables you to anticipate when the person will need to use the toilet, and share out the work of getting them there in time.

Toilet aids

Adaptations can be made to the bathroom and toilet area so that the person feels safe and secure while maintaining continence. Again, advice should be sought from an occupational therapist.

If mobility problems mean someone needs to use a commode rather than the toilet, staff should take care to respect the person's dignity, particularly if they have to share a room with others. Other people, including staff, should be actively discouraged from entering the room while the person is using the commode.

Take care also not to leave anyone on their own on the toilet (or in the bathroom) for long periods of time. Staff should be at hand to reassure or assist if required.

Constipation

Constipation is a common problem for people with learning disabilities, since it is associated with impaired mobility, poor diet and inadequate toilet arrangements. So keep people moving (see Chapter 16), help them use the toilet when they need to and in privacy, make sure they have enough to drink and plenty of foods that are rich in fibre – "roughage" which makes faeces softer, bulkier and easier to pass (see the list of foods on p.111).

Faecal impaction (severe constipation)

Here constipation is so bad that it causes a blockage in the bowel, which can press on the bladder and cause incontinence of urine. It is also a common cause of faecal incontinence, which may be mistaken for diarrhoea, as liquid faeces leak around the solid blockage.

Infection control

Dealing with incontinence not only requires sensitivity and tact but also scrupulous attention to hygiene. Many illnesses, some of them serious, are spread through contact with urine or faeces.

First help the person clean themselves up, using disposable wipes and/or soap and water, and deal with soiled clothing (handling as little as possible). They will need to wash their hands, and you should wash your own hands with scrupulous care afterwards.

Any spillages on floor or furniture should be cleaned up thoroughly, using rubber gloves and a solution of bleach or household disinfectant. Cloths must be sterilised afterwards in a bleach solution. Take care that floor/toilet cloths do not come into contact with face cloths or dish cloths.

Your service should have written guidelines on practice in this area.

Conclusion

Feeding, bathing and toileting are central to good care and a major way in which we can express our respect for the people we support. Services often look "busy", but if we are rushing people through meals, leaving the bathroom door open or failing to deal sensitively with incontinence, we are missing important opportunities to build people's self-esteem and enrich their day-to-day lives.

Points to remember

Help with eating and drinking. Ask yourself:

1. Has the person had the opportunity to use the toilet?
2. Are their clothes dry and comfortable?
3. Are they sitting in an upright position?
4. Is the table at the correct height so the person can reach and see their food?
5. Are they with other people?
6. Has the person contributed to the meal, its choice or preparation?
7. Does the staff team know the person's likes and dislikes?
8. Are the mealtimes flexible?
9. Does anyone have difficulty chewing?
10. Do you need any aids or equipment?

Help with personal care. Ask yourself:

1. Is the bathroom warm?
2. Have you both got everything you need?
3. Do other staff members know where you are so you won't be disturbed?
4. Do you need any aids or equipment?
5. Have all the risks been identified and the person consulted on the amount of support they need?

Incontinence. Ask yourself:

1. Has it just begun?
2. How often is it happening?
3. Has the person been seen by a GP to rule out any medical reasons, such as a urinary tract infection?

CHAPTER 15

Sexuality

Hilary Brown

• Sexuality covers a wide range of our feelings and behaviour • Intimate contact that calls for tact and delicacy – imagine how you would feel • Balancing rights and risk – making difficult decisions • Working as a team, consulting together • Confidentiality • Sex education that covers both facts and feelings

Like everyone else, people with learning disabilities have sexual feelings and a right to express them. As a carer, you are likely to be involved in caring for people intimately in a way which means you will be aware of their sexuality; you will probably be involved in helping people to learn appropriate behaviour, and in helping them to make relationships. You may need to step in if someone with learning disabilities is being taken advantage of, and you may also need to offer people support if their sexual relationships don't work out the way they would like, if they are lonely, or not able to find a partner.

A range of feelings

First of all we should define what we mean by sexuality. It doesn't only mean "having sex" but includes a much wider range of feelings about ourselves – how we feel about being a man or a woman, what kind of relationships we have and enjoy, sensual pleasures like eating and drinking, soaking in a hot bath and eating chocolates, our health and fitness, our appearance and the way we present ourselves to others. All these things are central to our feelings of self esteem and confidence.

Close contact

Caring brings you into contact with people in an intimate way. There are not many jobs where, within a few days, you will be expected to take someone of the opposite sex to the toilet or bath them. You may not be used to seeing people with no clothes on, and feel embarrassed or awkward. Experienced carers get used to it and even get a bit blasé so you may need to ask for help from your colleagues. They will probably have forgotten how they felt!

The way you do these tasks is very important to the self respect and self esteem of the people you are caring for. It is very important that you respect their cultural rules and traditions about how such care is given. For example, women from Asian cultures will not expect to be given personal care by a man, some people prefer showering to bathing, and so on. Ask them or their relatives for more information so that you do not disrupt the pattern of care the person is used to.

If you imagine needing help with toileting yourself you can see how delicate a role it is. On the one hand you don't want someone who is too obviously uncomfortable, so that you feel awful if, for example, you have an erection, or your period starts, or you make a smell, but on the other hand you don't want someone who goes over the top in trying to put you at your ease by making jokes and comments. You certainly wouldn't want someone to make you feel that you are a nuisance or abnormal; in fact one of the most reassuring things you can say to someone to get you both through an embarrassing moment, is "It's all right, it happens to the best of us!"

Because of your role as a carer you will inevitably have to deal with erections, periods, wet dreams and masturbation. Because your job is also to help people socially you will be aware of relationships and people's hopes and disappointments in their sexual and romantic lives. All of these situations demand sensitivity on your part about what is right, not for you, but for the person concerned. Making decisions about sexuality is difficult because we tend to be brought up with strong views about what we should and shouldn't do. Surveys show that people always think that what they do is "normal" and that what other people do is odd! You may feel that masturbation is wrong, but it is not your job to impose this view on the people you are working with. Instead you should help them to find an appropriate place so that they are not embarrassed or embarrassing to others. Similarly, you might not agree with homosexuality but your job will not be to stop the person you work with from having same-sex relationships; your job will be to help him or her to decide for themselves about the relationships and sexual activities which feel right for them.

Rights and risks

People with mild and moderate learning disabilities have the same rights, although they do not enjoy the same opportunities, to enter into sexual relationships as anyone else. People with *severe* learning disabilities are deemed not to be able to give their consent to enter into sexual relationships because the law is designed to protect them from exploitation. But usually such matters do not come to court and the law is not invoked where two people who care for each other are having a relationship.

In this situation you will have to decide as a staff team whether they are willing partners or if either one of them is being hurt or used. You will need to think about how much they understand about sexual behaviour and its possible consequences (pregnancy and sexually transmitted diseases for example) as well as look at the balance in the relationship to see if both people want it, as opposed to a situation in which one person is forcing him/herself on the other, or taking advantage by getting them to spend all their money, or using them and then going away. You will need to be particularly sensitive to the possibility of violence in a relationship, or emotional bullying. But making such decisions is not easy – you have to steer a course between being so protective that the person has no chance to learn from their mistakes, and too "laid back", allowing things to get out of their control.

Always consult

The golden rule is not to make such decisions on your own. Always consult with your colleagues and reach a consensus between you so that you can be consistent with the people concerned and also so that you can act as a sounding board for each other. In any staff team there will be a spread of opinion and experience, so that together you can make a more balanced decision than one person acting alone. You may do this in the context of individual planning or you may use staff meetings to explore what is happening.

Because you are not just a "friend" to the people you work with, you have a duty to discuss relationship issues with the staff team or with your manager. This would be especially important if you thought someone was being abused, but it is also important if you need to discuss how best to help people in relationships they want to continue.

Confidentiality

This means that there are different rules about confidentiality from those you might have with your friends. This issue is not only *who* you talk to about private matters which people with learning disabilities have confided in you, but *how* you talk to others.

Firstly, you must not talk about people outside of work, just as you would not like your private matters to be spread around. Secondly, you must share any information with the other people who are responsible for helping the person. This is partly for the benefit of the client, but also for your own protection so that you do not get involved yourself without checking out what other people think is the best course of action.

Lastly, it is important that where there are potentially risky situations the whole team is involved in making decisions, and where there are ongoing problems like difficult sexual behaviour, you get proper professional help from a psychologist or social worker before the person gets themself into trouble.

Social opportunities

So far we have talked more about intervening to stop something happening. The other side of your job is to be actively involved in making things happen for people. By this, I do not necessarily mean acting as a matchmaker

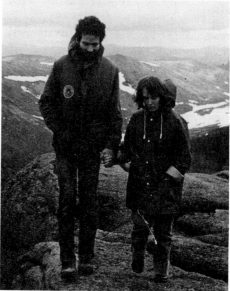

Photo: Mencap

You will be aware of relationships, people's hopes and disappointments, and you need to be sensitive to what is right, not for you, but for the person concerned.

but helping people to get a positive sense of themselves as men or women. Helping people with their clothes and appearance, fixing opportunities for them to have a good social life, to go dancing, to meet other people of their age, to go on holidays with a wider group of people. This is particularly important where people are living in small group homes and may end up quite isolated without some definite planning on the part of staff. Sometimes people who moved out of hospital were allowed to lose touch with friends and lovers they had known for ages, while people who have lived at home may not have had chance to develop friendships away from the watchful gaze of their parents.

Sex education

Sex education is another important way of being positive. Many of us had to start our sexual relationships without proper information or support. People with learning disabilities find it especially difficult to get hold of accurate and unbiased information. Their peers may not know much either so that they cannot make use of informal channels of information, and sometimes the contradictory images and messages which come through advertising and television need some deciphering.

Parents may also find it difficult to talk about sexuality to their sons and daughters with disabilities, not only because of the embarrassment which tends to surround such conversations but from not knowing what they should say and how to help their son or daughter understand. They may feel that it is best to avoid the issue because they do not want to raise something which they cannot deal with, or to arouse expectations which they feel could cause pain to their sons and daughters.

As a result parents often seem to voice protective feelings while staff tend to take on a more campaigning role around sexuality. Both are important and it is unfortunate that sexuality tends to turn into a battleground. It needs skill and tolerance on the part of staff to listen to the uncertainties which parents voice, to their own underlying grief which may be triggered for example in acknowledging that they will not have grandchildren, or the practical difficulties of their ongoing role as carers when other parents of their age have let go of their child-rearing responsibilities.

Don't label

In the face of such emotions it is important that staff do not become glib, or dismissive of parents, labelling them "overprotective" or saying that they cannot "let go". The truth is that parents are involved for life whereas staff come and

go, parents are moreover emotionally involved while staff can see the person's sexuality as an "issue". Also, staff can compare this person's problems and aspirations with those of other people with learning disabilities, where parents will only have their other sons and daughters as a reference point and will be brought face to face with comparisons which they may find very painful.

Disappointments

People with learning disabilities will also pick up on the ways in which their lives are different from other people's. They will be aware that their opportunities to find a partner or to have children, for example, are not the same as their brothers or sisters. If they have visible handicaps they will have had to manage other people's embarrassing stares and questions. They may have low self esteem when comparing themselves with others or with people they see on television and in magazines. Above all they may have failed time and time again to get their feelings and hopes to be taken seriously. It isn't that people deliberately avoid issues or tell reassuring lies, but that it is easier and sometimes seems kinder to avoid these things.

But people with learning disabilities need space to explore for themselves what their options are as men and women with disabilities. They often have very realistic expectations but may sometimes want to acknowledge that they would have liked things to have been different. Often for example, we get caught up in cheery conversations about a wedding in the family without allowing the person to say that they wish it had been them rather than their "luckier" sister or brother who was getting married.

Staff have a difficult balance to maintain. You need to steer a course between being so gloomy that you fail to support people in going out and getting what they want, and loudly championing their rights and standing up for them to the extent that you are insensitive to their more painful feelings of loneliness or inadequacy.

Sex – facts and feelings

Sexuality can be a very positive force in our lives, but it also heightens people's sense of vulnerability and hurt.

A good sex education programme would therefore include facts and feelings. It would present information but also allow people to apply what they learn to their own situation and face up to their real, rather than idealised experiences and hopes.

Materials have been developed to cover the main points, for people with both mild and severe learning disabilities. These are helpful because there is no point in "beating about the bush", and sensitive pictures help you to get the message across. These packs are very different from pornography – they are designed to inform rather than titillate. Many services have policies which say that pornography should not be introduced by staff, because although it may show actions which are explicit and which could be seen as educational, there is often an underlying inequality about the "poses" and imagery which is not appropriate.

Sex education is best carried out on a planned basis and agreed with the whole staff team. You should work with another member of staff so that you can constantly get feedback about how much people are understanding and what are appropriate goals for each individual. As in all work involving sexuality, for your own protection as well as for the benefit of those you work with, you should always seek the advice and agreement of your colleagues and manager before you begin.

The curriculum might cover:

- body parts
- appropriate sexual language
- masturbation
- relationships with the opposite sex
- same sex relationships
- contraception and safer sex
- parenthood
- menstrual hygiene
- menopause
- other sexual health issues
- assertiveness: when to say yes and when to say no
- sexual abuse
- appropriate behaviour in public.

But there is no such thing as a standard curriculum as people vary so much. Some people may understand all the basic facts of life and nuances of behaviour, whereas for others more limited aims will be set – such as helping them to behave appropriately in public, or to protect themselves.

Wherever possible the carer should use the language and terminology which the person with learning disabilities introduces into the conversation, and gear what they are saying to that person's level of understanding (see Chapter 5 on Communication). There is no point in getting into complicated biological explanations if more basic information is all the person can understand.

Training and support

As well as regular discussions with your colleagues, you can ask for training to enable you to explore what your views are and get comfortable talking about sex and sexual issues. This might be organised by your own agency or by an organisation such as the Family Planning Association, who run courses specifically for care staff working with people with learning disabilities. You should also have a policy or guidelines about how to approach sexual matters with the people you are caring for: these act as a safeguard for you as well as for your manager. Such guidelines will not force you to do anything which you don't approve of but they should also make clear what the values of your organisation are and how they want you to approach the decisions and judgements you will face.

Your example

Because sexuality is an important part of the environment – remember your *working* environment is the *living* environment for the people you are caring for – it is important that the relationships which they see around them at work are respectful and good natured. You have a right as a worker not to be harassed at work and it is important that you stick up for yourself and, by implication, for the people you are caring for. If you are worried about sexual harassment at work and cannot get help within your establishment you could speak to a more senior manager, or if you work in a privately registered home, to the Homes Inspector.

One situation you may have to face is the problem of people you are caring for developing a "crush" on you. This puts you in as difficult position. Should you be very clear and risk being unkind or "play them along" in a light hearted way? It is difficult not to feel flattered by such attention, but this should not influence you in deciding what is best for you to do. Again the best way forward is to consult your colleagues so that they can help to defuse the situation. Crushes illustrate the problem people with learning disabilities have of finding suitable and available partners, and also is a reminder of how important a role you play in their lives as a member of care staff. While your social life may be full, you may be the highlight of someone else's day, and that is always a difficult situation to manage.

Another dilemma which may arise is to what extent you involve the people you are caring for in your own social life and relationships. We have seen in Chapter 10 that sharing your social interests and friends can work to the benefit of the people you are caring for, but you might also need to keep some boundaries.

If, for example, you have a boyfriend or girlfriend who visits you at work or involves themselves in social activities you will have to be sensitive to the way this is perceived by the people you work with. They may enjoy the extra social contact; on the other hand they may feel you are distracted by your friend's presence, or feel that you are flaunting your good fortune in front of them. As with so many of these issues there is no right or wrong answer, just the need to be aware of the effect your relationships, values and views have on the people you are caring for.

A vital part of life

We have come a long way towards creating opportunities for people with learning disabilities to enjoy their own bodies and relationships. In the old hospitals, wards used to be segregated and privacy non-existent. Sensual pleasures like hot baths and nice clothes were unthought of, and people were often regarded as children throughout their lives.

It is important that we keep this barren picture in mind as we struggle to make good decisions in new services. It might be easy to think that skirting round sexual issues would save time and effort, but the way we feel about our bodies and relationships is so central to our lives and to the lives of the people with learning disabilities with whom we work, that we cannot give up on them. Sexuality is at the heart of an "ordinary" life, and it is up to us to keep it there.

Points to remember

1. Everyone is "sexual" and has a right to enjoy their body and make relationships as far as they are able. Men and women with learning disabilities may need your support to do this.

2. "Sexuality" isn't just about sex, it is about how people feel about themselves and others.

3. In offering intimate care to people through tasks such as bathing and toileting you will need to respect the person's cultural values and dignity.

4. You may have to deal with things which are embarrassing to you and to the person you are caring for.

5. People with learning disabilities are entitled to protection from situations which they do not want or cannot understand. In relationships, talk together about whether both partners are consenting, and if you think they are able to understand enough about sex to give consent.

6. ALWAYS consult your colleagues if you are in doubt about a relationship. Don't gossip but do consult.

7. Respect parents' views and feelings. Remember they are more involved than you and their caution may be justified.

8. Plan sex education and counselling sessions with your manager and colleagues. Make sure they know what you are doing, and make use of published teaching resources which are clear, respectful and explicit. Remember to gear your teaching to the needs of specific individuals.

9. Listen to painful feelings such as disappointment and loneliness, as well as more optimistic and hopeful feelings. Everyone feels down sometimes and the last thing they need is false cheerfulness.

10. If you are interested, get further training for yourself to increase your confidence and comfort in talking about sexual issues.

Further reading and contacts

Family Planning Association, Education Unit, 27-35 Mortimer Street, London W1N 7RJ.

For information on sexual abuse contact **Dr Ann Craft**, The University of Nottingham, Faculty of Medicine, Department of Mental Handicap, Floor E, South Block, University Hospital, Nottingham NG7 2UH, and

Hilary Brown, Centre for Applied Psychology of Social Care, Hut 1, Beverley Farm, University of Kent at Canterbury, Canterbury, Kent CT1 7LZ.

New Lifestyles for People with Learning Difficulties (including an extension cards set specifically on sexual issues) available from Pavilion Publishing (Brighton) Limited, 42 Lansdowne Place, Hove, East Sussex BN3 1HH.

Craft A and members of the Nottinghamshire Severe Learning Disabilities Sex Education Project 1991. *Living your Life: a Sex Education and Personal Development Programme for Students with Severe Learning Disabilities*, LDA, Department G, Duke St, Wisbech, Cambs PE13 2A3.

Fit for life (1983). Macmillan Education, Basingstoke.

Living your life, LDA (address above).

Brook Advisory Centres (1987). *Not a child any more.* A sex education programme for older teenagers and adults. Brook Advisory Centres, Birmingham.

Craft, A. et al (1983). "A Health and Sex Education Programme: Curriculum and Resources". Chapter in Craft, A. and Craft, M. (eds) *Sex Education and Counselling for Mentally Handicapped People*, Costello Press, Tunbridge Wells, Kent.

Craft, A (in press). *Sex Education for Students with Learning Disabilities: a guide to resources.* Available from Dr A. Craft, address above.

Dixon, H (1988) *Sexuality and Mental Handicap: An Educator's Resource Book*, LDA, Cambridge.

Dixon H and Craft A (1992). *Picture Yourself.* Four packs of illustrated cards, LDA (address above).

CHAPTER 16

Movement and lifting

Barbara Ogden

• Why it is so important to stay active • Everyday activities, self care and household chores keep people fit • Walking aids and wheelchairs - how to choose and use them • Guidelines for safe lifting

One of the most difficult tasks facing care staff is to maintain a balance between offering an appropriate level of help and encouraging the development of someone's own abilities and skills. Many tasks can be very time consuming – bathing, dressing, toileting, for example. It often seems quicker and easier for care staff to do the task for the person rather than finding enough time to work with them so that they can accomplish the task themselves.

Staff shortages, sickness, annual leave, household chores, crisis management, individual planning, team meetings, training, shopping, cooking, cleaning - all these things must be dealt with in the course of a day's work, so it is not surprising that care staff often fall back on the quickest way of doing something rather than the best way for the person with learning difficulties.

It is vital though that people are given as much opportunity as possible throughout the day to maintain and develop their physical skills: sitting, standing, walking, transferring independently, manoeuvring a wheelchair or climbing stairs for example, because any reduction in level of activity will reduce their independent mobility, increasing the need for physical assistance from care staff.

For everyone, activity is vital to maintain body functions. Any loss of activity, or a period of inactivity, will affect all the major systems of the body such as the heart, lungs, bones, muscles and joints, and reduce someone's overall level of fitness. If they become more dependent on care staff or carers for assistance there is also a psychological impact - loss of motivation, confidence and reduced self esteem. The person with learning disabilities has little or no motivation to accomplish a task themselves if they know it will be performed more quickly and with less effort by care staff. This gradual erosion of confidence and self esteem coupled with the loss of physical skills and increased dependence on others, leads to them becoming more "disabled" and requiring more care:

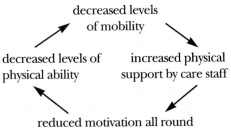

decreased levels of mobility

decreased levels of physical ability

increased physical support by care staff

reduced motivation all round

So take every opportunity to let people do what they can: don't lift them in and out of bed if they are able to stand and take weight through their legs; don't wheel them to the toilet in a wheelchair if they are able to walk, and so on.

The effects of inactivity

Muscles and joints

As we grow older we all tend to become less active, and this can affect the amount of calcium in the bones. One of the effects of reduced calcium is brittleness (osteoporosis). This means, for example, that a fall in an older person is much more likely to cause a fracture than in a younger person. One of the most effective ways of maintaining calcium in the bones and preventing further loss is by encouraging weight bearing through the bones – in the case of the legs by standing and walking.

Immobility causes muscles to weaken through disuse and the joints to stiffen. As you get older your joints begin to suffer from wear and tear which can lead to pain, stiffness and swelling (osteoarthritis).

Circulation

The more active you are the more vigorously the heart pumps to circulate blood round your body. Immobility and inactivity causes the circulation to become sluggish and allows blood to pool in veins (varicose veins). Tissue fluids may also be less quickly cleared through the system, leading to swelling, particularly in feet and ankles.

Without regular movement the body becomes less able to adapt quickly to changes in position, so for example if someone rises quickly from a chair they may become light headed, dizzy and unsteady (due to a sudden fall in blood pressure). This should be borne in mind when helping someone to stand up or get out of bed; you should allow time for them to regain their balance and equilibrium.

Pressure areas

Pressure maintained on an area of the body for extended periods of time, through sitting or lying too long in one position, will eventually lead to skin and tissue breakdown, and the development of pressure sores. These can be very difficult and slow to heal, and if they become infected can be life threatening, requiring major surgery and tissue repair to enable healing.

So it is very important to give people motivation and help to move about, getting up from a chair regularly and not spending too long in any one position. If someone is unable to move themselves, because of disability or illness, you will need to change their position regularly by lifting. Someone who is confined to a wheelchair should have been taught to lift themselves off the seat by taking their weight on their arms briefly but regularly; they may need reminding to do this. Aids such as foam or gel cushions, or sheepskins, can be helpful: ask a district nurse, occupational therapist, physiotherapist or your local Disablement Services Centre for advice.

Respiration

If someone is inactive this also affects the respiratory system, which becomes less effective in clearing secretions and maintaining full air entry to the lungs, which can predispose a person to chest infections and in the older person even pneumonia.

Keeping people active

The simplest way of maintaining mobility is by maintaining or increasing levels of activity. This does not necessarily mean encouraging people to exercise, attend keep fit classes and so on. Start by ensuring that people remain active throughout the day, taking part in a variety

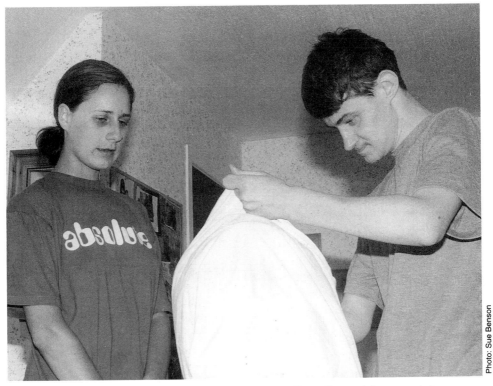

Housework – changing bed linen for example – is an excellent all-round fitness activity.

Photo: Sue Benson

of household chores and activities (see Chapter 8). Housework is an excellent all-round fitness activity: dusting, hoovering, washing floors, making beds - all encourage muscle strength and joint range, increasing general fitness. If someone is physically disabled and uses a wheelchair, there are still plenty of household activities they can share, such as dusting, clearing tables, cooking.

As people become older their increased age should be taken into account when sharing out household tasks, but old age does not mean that the person should spend all day sitting in front of the TV –this is a recipe for deterioration in both physical and mental health and wellbeing.

Regular exercise is very important. Walking is one of the best and most important forms of exercise available, and should be encouraged whenever possible. Swimming is another activity which exercises all body systems and increases levels of fitness. Other activities such as bowling, trampolining, riding, keep fit, weight training and gardening are also useful and enjoyable.

Walking aids

When does someone need a walking aid? If they have:

- an unsteady gait
- increasing weakness and joint stiffness
- pain or discomfort on walking
- a tendency to lose their balance when walking outdoors or on uneven ground
- frequent falls.

Points to consider:
1. The space available: is there room for a walking frame?
2. The person's ability to use the aid appropriately.

3. Is it to be used indoors/outdoors?

4. Will it need to be transported in a car or on public transport?

5. Are there stairs to be negotiated?

Walking aids are normally supplied free of charge on the NHS after proper assessment by a physiotherapist. Some GPs and community occupational therapists may supply aids. The advice of such a qualified person should always be sought before buying a walking aid for anyone.

Sometimes it is necessary to try several different types of aids with the user before deciding which is the safest and most appropriate aid for that person.

Walking sticks

These can be wooden or metal, fixed height or adjustable. Walking sticks should always be adjusted to the correct height for the user.

Sticks may be used singly or in pairs. When one stick is used it should normally be held in the hand opposite the weakest or most painful leg.

If the user has difficulty gripping the handle of an ordinary stick, a Fischer-type stick may be more appropriate. This has a moulded hand grip which is easier to grasp if you have poor hand function.

Walking frames

There are several types of walking frames:

1. Standard frame: (sometimes known as a Zimmer frame, but this is a trade name). These come in different sizes (small, medium, large) and can be fixed height or adjustable. They can also have a wide or narrow base; for most people using them in a domestic setting a narrow frame is best unless the person is particularly unsteady on their feet.

Like sticks, frames should be adjusted to the correct height for the user; they should not therefore be "communal", to be used by anyone.

2. Wheeled frames (rollators). These frames have small wheels at the front and are pushed along the ground rather than lifted up. They are useful for people who have poor balance, or who are unable to lift a frame forward with each step, perhaps due to weakness of the arms.

3. Gutter frames. These are taller and have "gutter" shaped supports for the forearms. The user leans on the frame and pushes it forward. They are used when someone needs a lot of support to walk, but as they are rather large, cumbersome and difficult to manoeuvre in confined areas, they are not ideal for use in an ordinary house.

Other aids

Other less usual aids include quadrupods (a stick with four feet), tripods (similar but with three feet) and crutches. Tripods and quadrupods are sometimes used if someone has a hemiplegia (paralysis of one side of the body) but are also quite cumbersome and have to be used correctly, or there is a danger of tripping over. Crutches are sometimes issued following a fracture or other leg injury; but they have to be correctly used and it is often simpler for the person to have a frame temporarily.

Safety and maintenance

1. An aid should always be adjusted by a qualified person such as a physiotherapist, to the right height for the person using it. Aids should not therefore be considered as available for use by other people resident in the same house, no matter how similar their needs may be.

In a house where several people have walking aids, discreet marking of the aid with a label or etching can be useful.

2. The rubber ferrules on the tips of sticks and frames should be checked regularly for wear. If someone leans heavily on the aid they can wear out remarkably quickly and should be replaced as necessary.

Ferrules can normally be obtained from the supplier of the aid, or bought from medical equipment suppliers or larger branches of chemist shops such as Boots.

3. The metal nuts and bolts which hold walking frames together can become loose over a period of time, and should be tightened up with a spanner.

4. If you are in any doubt about the safety of a walking aid, seek advice from a qualified person such as a physiotherapist, who can "condemn" an unsafe aid and supply a new one as required.

5. If someone no longer needs an aid because their mobility improves, please notify the agency who supplied it who will normally arrange for the aid to be collected. If it is in reasonable condition it can be cleaned and used for someone else.

Wheelchairs

Wheelchairs are normally supplied through the local Disablement Services Centre (DSC) at the request of an NHS doctor or therapist. Each health district falls within the catchment area of a DSC, which is responsible for the provision and maintenance of wheelchairs. Wheelchairs supplied through the DSC are on loan for as long as is necessary; they are not the property of the user and so should not be altered or modified in any way without the permission of the DSC.

Wheelchairs can also be bought privately, but assessment by a qualified therapist is vital to avoid an expensive mistake. Places such as the Disabled Living Foundation and Keep Able Centres have a wide range of chairs to try out and trained staff available to advise.

How to get a wheelchair

• If someone only needs a wheelchair for a very short time, one can sometimes be obtained on loan from a hospital, social services department or local branch of the Red Cross.

• If a wheelchair is needed for long term or permanent use, a request form needs to be completed by a doctor or therapist. Contact your local DSC for advice, or the person's GP.

It is very important that an assessment is undertaken by a suitably qualified person (usually a therapist) to determine the person's individual needs, the environment and circumstances in which the chair will be used, and the most appropriate type of chair to meet those needs.

Points to consider

1. Age and ability of the individual:
• Are they able to self-propel a chair or will they need to be pushed?
• Would they be able to operate a powered (electric) chair?
• Are special adaptations necessary to enable the person to use a wheelchair effectively?
• Would the individual be able to manoeuvre the chair safely, operate the brakes correctly, etc?

2. Where will the wheelchair be used?
• Indoors or outdoors?
• Does the chair need to be transported in the boot of a car?
• If for outdoor use, is the ground rough, uneven, hilly?
• If for indoor use, is there enough clearance through doorways, turning space in rooms and corridors? Are there deep pile carpets which make moving a wheelchair difficult? Will adaptations need to be made to the house to accommodate a wheelchair?
• Will the individual be spending long periods of time in the wheelchair?

Types of chair available

Manual – self-propelling: these have two large wheels at the back, which are used to propel the chair alone.

Push (transit) chairs: these have smaller wheels at the rear and cannot be propelled by the user who has to be pushed by an attendant.

Powered (electric): These can be for indoor use, indoor/outdoor use or outdoor use. The powered chairs for indoor/outdoor and outdoor use are not supplied through the DSC and have to be purchased privately.

Powered chairs for indoor use supplied by the DSC can be driven for short distances outdoors on the flat, but are unable to cope with slopes, kerbs or uneven ground.

Wheelchair safety and maintenance

It is vital that wheelchairs are kept well maintained for their safe operation. The following simple maintenance procedures should be undertaken by care staff at least weekly:

Tyres: Keep them well pumped up so that they feel firm to thumb pressure. Tyres must not be allowed to become flat as the brake mechanism will not then work. A bicycle pump is supplied with the chair when it is delivered, but many people find a foot pump easier. Minor punctures can be repaired using a bicycle repair kit.

Brakes: Check regularly to ensure they are working correctly. The brakes should work effectively even on a slope. The screws of the brake mechanism often work loose and should be tightened using a spanner. Remember that the brakes will not work properly if the tyres are flat or not pumped up enough.

Footrests: Check to ensure that they move freely and lock into position.

Canvas: The seat canvas and back rest canvas should be checked for rips or tears. If there is a tear, the approved repairers should be contacted to replace it.

Safety straps: Check for fraying, wear and tear, and that the clip works correctly.

Cleanliness: The chair should be regularly cleaned by wiping it down with a damp cloth. A dirty, poorly maintained chair does nothing to enhance the image of the user or assistant.

Repairs: Minor repairs such as tyre punctures or loose screws on brakes, may be carried out by care staff, but any more major repairs or alterations must be made by the Approved Repairer, who is authorised by the DSC to undertake wheelchair repair and maintenance. If you are unsure who your Approved Repairer is contact your local DSC.

Safe operation of wheelchairs

Care must be taken to ensure that the person is not at risk of injury when using a wheelchair.

Brakes: These should always be applied whenever the chair is stationary, and particularly when the user is transferring to and from the chair. It is the responsibility of care staff to ensure that the brakes are used correctly, whether by the wheelchair user or by care staff.

Footrests: Most chairs have footrests that can be removed or swung out of the way when not in use. It is very important that this is done when the user is transferring to and from the chair, as it is easy for them or their helper to catch their feet on the footrests, and fall. Footrests should be replaced or swung back to the correct position once the user is sitting correctly in the chair, and the wheelchair should not be pushed without the footrests being in position. Serious injuries have been caused by pushing a chair without footrests: feet and ankles can become trapped against kerbs, door frames etc.

Safety straps: These should always be used when supplied, or whenever the user is at risk of falling out of the chair, as they may be when travelling over rough ground or down a slope. If someone has difficulties with balance, extensor spasm, epilepsy etc, then they should have a safety strap. If you think someone needs a safety strap and hasn't got one, contact your local DSC for advice.

Comfort: Wheelchairs are not designed with comfort in mind, simply as a means of transportation. Unless they have a specialist seating system, for example a moulded seat contoured to fit the shape of the body, the individual should not be encouraged to sit for extended periods in the wheelchair. Most chairs are supplied with cushions when delivered (usually two-inch vinyl covered foam) and these should be used. If someone is vulnerable to pressure sores, has poor circulation, fragile skin, or is very thin and bony, then a pressure relieving cushion may be required. Contact your Disablement Services Centre, physiotherapist or occupational therapist for advice.

Pushing a wheelchair

This is hard work! It is particularly difficult if the ground is uneven or if there are many slopes or hills to negotiate. It is much easier if the tyres are kept well pumped up. There are tipping bars on the back of most wheelchairs to enable the chair to be tipped up to negotiate kerbs or steps, or to descend steep slopes.

Access

Wheelchair access is still poor in this country though efforts are being made to improve it where possible by installing lifts and ramps. If someone is denied access to a public building such as a shop, cinema or pub because it is inaccessible to someone with a physical disability, you should encourage them to write, or write on their behalf to the appropriate person, such as the manager of the shop or local councillors.

Transport

Motability: People receiving Mobility Allowance may make use of the Motability Scheme, to help towards the purchase of an adapted car, or powered wheelchair.

Dial-a-Ride: This scheme provides a door-to-door transport service for people who are unable to use existing public transport because of a disability. It cannot be used to take people to and from hospital appointments, or where local authorities provide transport.

RADAR: The Royal Association for Disability and Rehabilitation will advise on all aspects of disability, including access and transport. RADAR, 25 Mortimer Street, London W1N 8AB. Tel: 071 637 5400.

Points to remember

Activity, aids and wheelchairs

1. Ensure that people with learning disabilities are given time and support to maintain and develop physical skills, and make sure that any physical assistance offered is tailored to the needs and abilities of that individual.

2. Ensure that everyone has plenty of opportunity for regular exercise and physical activity.

3. Walking aids and wheelchairs should never be shared.

4. Regular cleaning, checking and maintenance of walking aids and wheelchairs is vital.

5. Never use a piece of equipment that is unsafe.

6. Remember that people's needs may change due to increasing age or health problems, and so regular reassessment of equipment is required.

Lifting

Correct lifting is a vital skill which must be learned and then practised regularly to ensure and maintain competence.

There is no one correct method of lifting so care staff should receive training in a variety of different techniques and methods, which can then be adapted to suit the various circumstances and situations which are encountered.

There are however some basic points which apply to any lift whether it is an object, a heavy load or a person. These basic principles should also be applied when assisting someone to transfer, or when pushing or pulling a heavy load, for example someone in a wheelchair.

The importance of correct lifting cannot be over-emphasised, as lifting any load will increase the stress placed on your body and also therefore the risk of damage or injury. See Figures 1 and 2 opposite and the guidelines for safe lifting on p.132.

It is important to be aware of your posture at all times and to move in ways which minimise the stresses and strains on your body. Poor posture and movement can become a habit, and if you repeat it often enough what you are doing gradually begins to feel "right" even though it may be causing increased stress and potential damage. Damage is more likely if the following factors are also present:

• twisting movements
• holding a position for a period of time
• repetitive movements
• jerky, uncoordinated movement.

Most people tend to think of back pain in terms of slipped discs, but this is actually rather an uncommon injury. Muscles, joints and ligaments can be pulled and strained, usually only to a minor degree which resolves itself quickly with rest, but if repeated strains occur over a period of time then more serious damage and therefore a significant "back problem" may occur.

The ageing process also causes wear and tear of the spinal joints between the vertebrae and as you get older the potential for injury increases. It is therefore vital to think about your back at all times, not only when lifting objects, to ensure that stress and strain is minimised.

Before you lift

Don't lift unless you have to. Assess the situation fully to decide if a lift is necessary and ensure that any available help or aid is used. Always ask yourself these questions before attempting a lift:

• Is this lift necessary?

• Is there any help available from other people, or aids such as hoists, lifting belts, transfer boards?

• Can the person to be lifted help in any way? For example can they take weight through their legs, in which case a transfer rather than a lift would be appropriate?

• Do you have the confidence and competence to undertake the lift safely and correctly?

• Can this person or thing be moved in any other way (wheeled on a trolley for example)?

Assess the surroundings:
• Is there enough space available or can more be made by moving furniture or objects out of the way?

• Is the area clear of any hazards such as spilt liquids, trailing electric cables, mats and rugs which can be tripped over, pets etc?

• Over what distance will the object/ person need to be carried? Ensure it is as short as possible.

Assess the lift

Load:
• How heavy is the load? Test it first before lifting.

• Is the load an awkward shape, large, soft, sharp edged, hot, cold etc?

• Are there any handles which could be used?

Person:
• Is the person able to understand and co-operate with the lift?

• What are the person's abilities; can they assist in any way?

• Is the person agitated or confused? If so, ensure that plenty of help is available.

• What shape and size is the person (tall, thin, heavy, round)?

• Are there any medical conditions that need to be considered, eg increased muscle tone, stiff joints, painful areas or areas of discomfort?

Assess your own abilities
• Are you fit and able to lift? Do you have any back or joint problems, muscle weakness?

• Are you pregnant? If so then you should avoid lifting any heavy load and extra care must be taken to ensure that any lifting is done correctly.

• Do you know which technique to use?

• Do you feel confident in using this technique?

If in any doubt about your ability to lift, get help

• Ensure that you are dressed appropriately for lifting with no tight or restrictive clothing, or unsteady shoes.

• Remove any jewellery which could become entangled or cause injury: rings, watches, necklaces, earrings etc.

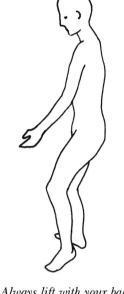

Figure 1: Always lift with your back straight, hips and knees bent, feet in a stable position. Lower yourself to the level of the load, but avoid going into a squatting position which is unstable and difficult to get up from.[1]

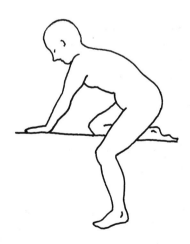

Figure 2. This is a good position to use when moving someone in bed. Place your knee on the bed for extra support and stability, and to avoid twisting your spine.[1]

Points to remember

Safe lifting

1. Always explain carefully what you are going to do, and ask the person to co-operate as much as possible.

2. Make sure the surrounding area is clear of any hazards such as spilt water or obstacles.

3. Make sure that the lift is over a short a distance as possible and that the destination – where you are lifting to – is prepared.

4. Know your own limitations. Do not attempt to lift or transfer alone if you do not feel confident that you can manage.

5. Stand as close as possible to the person/object to be lifted.

6. Make sure that you have a good firm comfortable hold of the person, and use the whole of your hand not just fingertips.

7. Keep your back straight, but do not hold yourself absolutely rigid.

8. Make sure you have your feet in a good safe position, with the leading foot pointing in the direction you will be moving in. Move your feet as you turn to avoid twisting the back.

9. Use hips, knees and body weight to lift. Lower yourself to the level of the object to be lifted and use the strong muscles in your legs to take the strain.

10. If two or three people are lifting, one should organise the lift so that everyone knows exactly what to do, and issue commands so that everyone lifts together.

11. Ensure that the lift chosen is comfortable for the person being lifted and that it does not cause undue strain on vulnerable joints such as painful stiff shoulders and hips.

12. If you are lifting to or from a wheelchair or other seat on wheels, ensure that the brakes are on and that footrests are out of the way. If there are no brakes, place chair against a wall or fixed object, and make sure it will not move while you lift it.

References

1. Based on examples given in Movement and Lifting for Carers, by Martin Hutchinson and Rosemary Rogers (Woodhead Faulkner, 1991). This book is recommended for further reading.

> Planning and preparation are as important as technique in ensuring that lifting is safely performed. But it is also vital that you receive practical training in lifting technique.

CHAPTER 17

How to get good health care

Helen Jeffery and Mike Higgs

• Why access to good health care is so important • Recognising signs and symptoms • Choosing and using your GP • Dental care • Screening

Good health care is one of the most influential factors in people's lives, affecting motivation, development and behaviour. We **all** have a right to good health care, from a variety of professionals and care staff in hospitals and the community. Studies have shown, however, that although people with learning disabilities have greater and more varied health care needs, they have often been given low priority.

The rapid development of community services has also meant that health professionals are suddenly faced with high expectations to provide comprehensive support, although many have limited skills and knowledge in the area of learning disability, and limited budgets.

So the carer – whether relative, advocate or member of care staff – has a very important role in raising awareness of the needs of the person with a learning disability, so that their doctor or dentist can treat them appropriately.

Health can be considered under two headings: physical health, relating to the workings of the body; and mental health, relating to the mind. The two are of course closely related, and when illness affects the body it is likely to change our behaviour in large or small ways. It is

therefore essential to check whether there are physical reasons for behaviour changes before deciding something is a mental health problem. Physical symptoms could otherwise remain undetected for long periods of time, especially in people who have severe learning disabilities or communication difficulties.

It is very important that we do not make easy or glib assumptions about signs of ill-health or particular symptoms by dismissing them as psychosomatic, or as someone exaggerating "for the sake of it". Sometimes, the person with a learning disability is unjustly labelled as lazy, awkward, a behavioural problem or of limited potential, when they may be held back by poor health, or experiencing pain. It may be that their symptoms could be relieved easily following medical examination and a course of treatment.

Recognising signs of illness

Most of us encounter common minor illnesses during our lives. We usually recognise them easily, by obvious physical symptoms such as coughs, sneezing, spots or rashes, and we can express in words and in some detail our sensations and the location of the problem. All this helps the professional make an accurate diagnosis. People with a learning disability find it difficult to convey their feelings in this direct way. They may be telling us that something is wrong through subtle, minor changes in actions or personality, or major changes in behaviour. Illness may be picked up through facial expressions, body language, changes in their routine, episodes of aggression, violence or antisocial behaviour. Incidents and actions often become even more extreme when people become frustrated at their inability to get others to understand their underlying problem.

Mental health is affected by both chemical reactions in the brain, and the person's reactions to situations, experiences and relationships. This is a specialist field often requiring counselling, therapy and medication (see Chapter 18). Prevention in this context means fostering environments where individuals feel safe and secure enough to enable them to express feelings and emotions. At the end of the day both the individual and the carer share the responsibility for maintaining good health helped by health education programmes, and community resources.

Prevention

Good health care always starts with prevention, wherever it is possible to take action to reduce the risks of illness or injury. Key factors are to be found in our daily routines, home environment, hygiene and safety standards, personal and sexual relationships. This incorporates our diet, exercise, personal hygiene, safety within daily living skills, knowledge of contraception and the use of immunisation programmes.

Observation

For the carer, observation and communication skills are especially important in relation to health - sometimes this could make the difference between what would have been a minor illness treated by a GP, and an emergency admission to hospital.

While it is often appropriate for the carer to provide treatment for what appear to be common illnesses, when these persist (for longer than three days) or recur they should be checked out, so that

---

CASE HISTORY: TIM

Tim, a 26 year old man with a history of eating rubbish, objects and items off the ground began to have episodes of diarrhoea. The care staff initially treated him with anti-diarrhoeal drugs, believing it to be a stomach upset caused by his eating habits. The condition persisted, and Tim became distressed and lethargic at times. He was rectally poking, smearing himself with faeces, continually stripping off, and pinching and biting fellow residents and care staff. They referred him to the doctor but despite stronger medication the condition persisted. An x-ray examination showed that the bowel was severely impacted; Tim was suffering from constipation and obstruction of the bowel, with the diarrhoea as an overflow from the condition.

The action taken by the staff in consultation with the GP was to:
i) Review his diet and fluid intake.
ii) Set up an intervention programme to reduce the incidence of eating rubbish.

Once the initial treatment had been started and the individual needs addressed, the diarrhoea stopped and all Tim's anti-social behaviours disappeared.

CASE HISTORY: SARAH

Sarah, a young lady in her early twenties, actively participated in most things and loved the company of others, but had sudden seemingly spontaneous changes of character. She would then become extremely moody, short tempered, reluctant to do things, and would hit out at fellow residents for no apparent reason. These episodes would last up to three or four days at a time.

On each occasion the staff took time to talk with her to see if anything was upsetting her. She could give no reason for her actions and was told that her behaviour to others was not acceptable.

On reviewing her personal file, staff noticed a pattern to the episodes: they occurred every month, a few days before her menstrual period. This was discussed with her key worker and doctor, who thought she might be suffering from premenstrual syndrome. She agreed to take medication prescribed by the doctor, which soon resulted in a marked improvement in all the symptoms.

assumptions are not made about the cause without consulting a medical practitioner. For example, "He's got a nasty cough" might be dismissed, "Because he smokes all the time". The person could have a chest infection unrelated to smoking, which needs and would respond to treatment.

For parents/relatives who care for individuals, noticing that something may be wrong is an easier task because they spend more time with the person and have a "global" picture of their unique habits, routines and characteristics.

For care staff working shifts the situation is less than ideal. It is like putting together a puzzle without the picture on the box. This requires individual staff to sort the pieces and work methodically to get the complete picture by gathering and sharing their understanding of an individual's needs, and making this accessible to those who will support the person. Such information gathering need not to be complicated. It could consist of a simple profile containing details of the persons likes/dislikes, individual routines, what usually motivates them and any forms of communication or expression which they used when they have been ill

in the past. Setting up such a record might initially be time-consuming but it will enable care staff to recognise potential problems in the early stages and provide immediate help and medical support.

Here are some common signs and symptoms which may indicate an underlying health problem:

PHYSICAL

Coughs, sneezing, rashes, spots, vomiting, diarrhoea, pallor, temperature, swelling, redness, sweats, difficulty in breathing, bleeding, discharges, bad breath.

BODY LANGUAGE

Grimacing, shivering, fidgeting, unable to sit still or settle, curling up in a ball, holding parts of the body continually, frowning.

ACTIONS/BEHAVIOURS

Head-banging, self-injurious behaviour, scratching, poking inside the mouth or rectum, screaming, crying, shouting, sitting on radiators or by fires, not wanting to get out of bed, short temper irritability, reluctance to join in activities, isolation, hitting out, constantly seeking attention and comfort.

SERVICES AVAILABLE IN THE AREA	Z's Health Centre	Dr X's Practice	Dr Y's Practice			Necessary services for the individual	Desirable services for the individual
Open surgery	✓	✓					✓
Appointments	✓		✓				✓
Wheelchair access	✓		✓			✓	✓
Well woman clinic							✓
Practice nurse	✓						
Community nurse							
Health visitor	✓	✓					
Chiropodist	✓		✓				✓
Women doctors	✓	✓					✓
Home visits	✓	✓	✓			✓	✓

It is useful to collect and compare information on all your local GP services.

Choosing a GP

Developing a good relationship with the general practitioners for the people you work with is essential as they will be your first "port of call" for medical help.

Available health services vary from area to area. It is therefore a valuable exercise, even if the person with learning disabilities already has a GP, to collect information about all of the services in the area and make sure they are getting the best care available, matching up what is on offer with the needs of each person. Depending on the ability and skill of the person with learning disabilities, this exercise could be done with them, their advocate, close relative or a friend. In making a choice of GPs it is important that you do not just make a block arrangement for all the people with learning disabilities living in a particular house. Having different GPs may help to ensure a personal approach. We have devised a chart (above) which can be used to help you see clearly which practice meets most of the needs of each person.

To interpret the chart, look at the services which are necessary for each person; in our example home visits and wheelchair accessibility are particularly important. Then eliminate from the chart the practices which do not provide these services. In this example Dr X's surgery is not suitable. Next, work out which of the remaining practices meets most of the needs you have identified. In our example, Z's Health Centre is the best.

Then the most appropriate doctor in this surgery should be approached – this choice should reflect the person's needs and preferences including considerations about their sex, ethnic origin and religion. If the doctor is confident that he/she will get consistent support from carers, they will usually agree to accept the person on their list.

Using your GP

To ensure the most effective use of your GP good communication is essential. This starts at home before an appointment is deemed necessary. Important information should be easily accessible to care staff in case they need it, and can be shared

APPOINTMENT RECORD CARD

NAME OF PERSON APPOINTMENT IS MADE FOR: *Tom Jones*

DATE	NAME OF PERSON MAKING APPOINTMENT	REASON FOR MAKING APPOINTMENT	DATE/TIME OF APPOINTMENT	NAME/ADDRESS OF DOCTOR
25/5 92	*Graham Thomson (support worker)*	*Tom has vomited three times today. The vomit is clear.*	*25/5/92* 5.30pm **10mins**	*Dr Charlie Baker New Road Clinic 6 New Road*
7/7 92	*Suzanne Jeffery Team Co-ordinator*	*Tom seems to have an ingrown toenail on the right foot. There is an infection.*	*10/7/92* 10.05am	*Dr Charlie Baker New Road Clinic 6 New Road*
10/9 92	*John Grame (advocate)*	*Tom has not been eating or sleeping well for one month.*	*30/9/92* 3.00pm **45mins**	*Dr P (referred by Dr X) Psychologist, Thornby Hospital, Mill Road*

You can make charts like this to keep all staff up to date; they are easy to fill in and refer to.

openly with people where possible. A general information sheet for each person could be helpful, whether they are seeing a health professional by themselves or to aid the memory of accompanying care staff. Such a sheet could actually be crucial when there is an emergency which puts everyone under stress, as people may then be unable to recall vital information.

The sheet should be set out to include the following information:

• Name, address and telephone number of both individual and their doctor
• Individual's date of birth, age, sex, cultural or ethnic background
• Next of kin and telephone number
• Special considerations to be taken into account while administering medical care
• Other important information including allergies
• Recent hospital visits, with dates and reasons
• Special medical instructions (if any) due to cultural or religious beliefs.

Making an appointment

When you think that a consultation with

the GP is necessary, think about what you need to say before speaking to the receptionist. Consider the following questions:

• Is it an emergency?
• Is a phone consultation enough?
• Is a home visit necessary? Why?
• Is a visit to the surgery necessary?
• Will a longer appointment be needed? (For example, due to communication difficulties, extreme distress or challenging behaviour).
• What appointment times are most suitable for the person?
• Is there any other information which would be helpful? (For example, the person doesn't like needles and can get very distressed or hit out if she sees one). It can help to write the answers to these questions down so that nothing is forgotten when you make the phone call.

Once the appointment has been made it is essential to log it correctly, so that other care staff know exactly what has happened and why. It is possible to do this in the following way on a appointment record card, as shown above.

Before a consultation make sure that the

EXAMINATION RESULTS CARD

NAME OF PERSON BEING EXAMINED: *Tom Jones*

DATE	DOCTOR'S NAME AND ADDRESS	RESULTS	ACTION NEEDED	NEXT APPOINTMENT
25/5/92	*Dr Charlie Baker New Road Clinic 6 New Road*	*Stomach bug*	**NO FOOD FOR 24 hrs** *Take medicine 3 x day until finished*	*None planned*

The information recorded on a chart like this is valuable to all care staff.

person has all their communication aids with them. This includes hearing aids, glasses, Makaton translations, and, photographs and pictures which the person with learning disabilities could point at, to enhance and assist their messages. If you accompany the person when they are meeting with the doctor, it is your role to enable and facilitate the person with learning disabilities to communicate what they can, in any way that they are able. However, it is sometimes necessary to elaborate on or correct important information, in a very respectful way, to assist the doctor to make an accurate diagnosis.

During or after the consultation make sure that any instructions from the doctor are carefully recorded. All care staff should then be told of these instructions. An example of a form, an examination results card, which can be used for this is shown above.

It is extremely important to administer and record medication correctly (see Chapter 18). You could develop your own system or seek advice from a community pharmacist. There are also aids from the chemist which could help care staff administer the right dose of medication at the right time. They come in a variety of forms but are usually plastic boxes with sections for different times in each day of the week.

Dental care

When dental care is mentioned many people automatically think only of their teeth, with little recognition to the important role of the gums in keeping everything in place. Along with this come many people's fears and anxieties of going to the dentist, because some people are so scared they only go in cases of emergency due to pain or discomfort. These beliefs are often passed on to others, with the result of encouraging poor oral hygiene, causing infections, gum disease and the loss of teeth.

For most of us the daily repetitive habit of cleaning our teeth is subconsciously incorporated within our routine, on getting up, going to bed, after meals and so on, and happens at least once a day. Even if we occasionally break this routine, we remember to clean them later without too much damage to our teeth and gums.

For people who have a learning disability the responsibility for good oral hygiene is often left to the carer, whether that means actually physically doing it for them or supporting them in personal programmes to enable them to do it independently. Both require consistency and monitoring, as we should not just be satisfied with frequency of teeth cleaning but how well it is done. It is also important to stress that individuals who do not have

BASIC DENTAL CARE PLAN			
For a person:	*WITH TEETH*	*WITHOUT TEETH*	*WITH DENTURES*
ORAL HYGIENE	Daily brushing with toothpaste, morning and evening. Dental floss when possible.	Massage gums with a soft toothbrush and dental gel.	Soak dentures overnight in denture cleaner and massage gums with a soft toothbrush and dental gel.
CHECK UPS	Minimum of every six months.	At least yearly.	Every year.
DIET	Attention to be paid to general diet, especially to the amount of sugary foods and sweets.		

A dentist's recommendations for minimum dental care.

teeth require as much care and attention as those who do.

It must be remembered that preventative measures are better than cures, and good dental care and oral hygiene can reduce the risks of dental problems. The effects of poor dental care can delay development of or reduce verbal communication, because infections or poorly fitted dentures have made speech painful. Certain medicines which people have to take on a regular basis can have side effects affecting the gums. In this case a higher level of dental care, advice and visits to the dentist or hygienist, may be needed.

Screening

Screening plays a significant role in preventive medicine. It is a way of detecting illnesses or conditions before they have a serious effect on our lives. These problems can then sometimes be addressed with the minimum of disruption to our lives. We all have rights to these screening services. The tests which are available to us will depend on our family history, our present condition, our sex and the area that we live in.

People with learning disabilities have the same rights of access to screening as anyone else, but they will not be able to take up their right of access unless they know what exists and are informed of the benefits of undergoing screening. This is very difficult because people are at different levels of understanding. We appreciate that there can be many hurdles, but we believe that where possible it is the care assistant's role to:

• Find out what screening could be available to that person.
• Educate and inform people about these opportunities and the consequences of both being and not being screened.
• Offer the informed choice.
• Assist and support people through the screening process.
• Help people with learning disabilities monitor and review their health and any medication given as a result of tests.

People with no formal way of communicating, or who do not seem to understand the situation, should also be offered these services but you may want to talk about your approach with their advocate, social worker, close friend or family member, and you will have to take a more active part in the decision making process on their behalf.

The following tests are commonly available for certain groups of people.

Find out whether these tests are appropriate for the people you support.

General screening
• Hearing test. Do this regularly (see Ch.6).
• Eye test.
• Cholesterol level tests.
• Chest x-rays.
• Blood pressure tests.
• Blood tests to check level of immunisation against Rubella, Polio, Hepatitis B.

Women
• Breast examinations.
• Cervical smear tests.
• Other tests for women using the contraceptive pill. Usually blood pressure and weight checks every six months.

Men
• Screening for prostate problems.

People who are diagnosed as having Down's syndrome:
• Thyroid function.
• Antlanto-axial instability/dislocation.

People from a West Indian Culture:
• Sickle Cell Disease.

This is by no means an exhaustive list but it will give you an idea of some issues to be aware of.

Community resources

There are times when people cannot use conventional health resources, or they require a more specialised service to meet their individual needs. There are services which span a variety of different aspects of health care, from professionals providing home visits to attendance at specific clinics. Access to and availability of resources varies from region to region. In most cases people can be referred by a GP, dentist or community nurse.

A useful point of reference for information is your local Community Team for People with Learning Disabilities (CTPLD), some of which may still be called Community Mental Handicap Teams (CMHT), who should be aware of local resources. Here are a few examples of services which may be available:
Well Woman Clinics
Community Health Units offering specialist services in dentistry, chiropody, ophthalmics and audiology
Community nurses
Occupational therapists
Physiotherapists
Health Promotion Teams

Conclusion

Good health care requires thoughtful planning and collaboration between care staff and local services. It relies on care staff working with people with learning disabilities to get the best out of the health service and on their working with health care professionals to make sure they can deliver the best service they know how. Providing information and acting as a "bridge" is an important contribution which care staff can make to better health and a more comprehensive health service for people with learning disabilities.

Points to remember

1. Don't rely on one GP for all your residents – choose a GP who will suit each individual.
2. Be on the lookout for signs or signals of illness. Remember changes of mood or behaviour could indicate pain.
3. Prepare for doctor's appointments – make sure you have the right information to hand.
4. Keep a record of symptoms, appointments and instructions from the doctor.
5. Help the person communicate with the doctor, and help the doctor communicate with the person you are supporting.
6. Don't forget dental care!

CHAPTER 18

Medical matters

David Brooks

• How medicines act in the body • The importance of timing, and giving medication strictly according to instructions • Routines that help • Medicines policy • Can a person self-administer their drugs? • Consent to treatment • Special medical needs – older age, epilepsy, mental health

We have seen in the last chapter that care staff have an important role to play in gaining access to good health care for people with learning disabilities, through the use of local doctors, clinics, dentists and hospitals. In this chapter we will focus on the role of care staff to follow up on the advice of other professionals; to see that medicines are given as they should be; to watch out for symptoms or side effects; to take note of common illnesses and conditions to which people with learning disabilities are vulnerable; and to work together with the other people involved in caring about and for the person's health.

Taking medicines

Taking medicine is a daily event for many people with learning disabilities, so it is important for care staff to understand how medicines act and how they can be safely administered. Usually this means in practice following your doctor or pharmacist's instructions, but knowing why you are doing something can help you to get it right.

The effect of a medicine will vary from individual to individual. It will depend on:

• what other drugs the person is taking and how these interact

• their general health and physical state

• the "route" of administration – for example whether swallowed as a tablet or applied as an ointment

• psychological factors, such as whether they believe the drug will make them better, or if they have had "bad" medicines in the past.

Thus the same dose prescribed to different people with the same disorder will have different outcomes and care staff have an important part to play in helping the doctor to monitor this and adapt the medication accordingly.

Drugs are given differently depending on individual needs and preferences, the organs they are designed to affect, and the best way for them to be absorbed into the body. Taking medicine on an empty stomach (unless it is an irritant to the stomach) will usually be the best way of ensuring quick absorption, whereas taking medicine after a meal will slow down the process. Remember alcohol is a drug and the same rules apply! Diarrhoea can also impair absorption, as can vomiting or other stomach upsets. This is the reason why women taking the contraceptive pill are advised to take other precautions if they have had any such sickness.

Some medicines are given in a way which bypasses the stomach altogether:
• as rectal or vaginal suppositories,
• under the tongue, or
• injected directly into the bloodstream.

The doctor will know how quickly and effectively the medicine can reach where it is needed. As care staff it is vital to follow instructions and to ask for clarification if you are unsure.

Timing is vital

It is not only the route of medication which is important, but also the intervals at which it is taken, and the timing. The doctor will need to understand the person's normal daily pattern of sleeping, waking, eating and going to the toilet, in order to prescribe medicines which will have the desired effect.

Taking a course of medicine is quite different from having the odd paracetamol when we have a headache. Dosage at intervals is necessary, often to keep a regular supply of the chemical in the body or to perform a particular function. If a medicine is given once a day the timing may depend on its purpose. It may, for example, be desirable to give water tablets in the morning to remove fluid which has accumulated in the night causing breathlessness or swollen ankles. If the same drug were given at night it could cause incontinence and distress. Some drugs make people tired while others might make them wakeful, so catching up on a missed dose needs to be considered very carefully.

Medicines given more than once a day tend to be given at meal times for ease of remembering and to make sure they are absorbed steadily into the bloodstream. However this might be too close together

for some medicines, such as antibiotics, and might leave too long a period overnight allowing the blood level to fall too low and the medicine be ineffective. It could also lead to unacceptably high levels in the daytime, which might cause side effects (this is a particular concern in the treatment for epilepsy). Some new medicines have "sustained release" mechanisms which regulate the release of the active ingredients over a twelve hour period. Obviously it is important that care staff check out instructions accurately to be sure they know what "three times a day" really means.

Some drugs are prescribed on the basis that they should only be given when required (for example, if someone has a seizure, or if they have a sudden migraine). The abbreviation often used for "as required" is "prn". Make sure you have clear guidance for deciding when you should give these drugs, and limits on the amount and frequency of doses. This is especially important where drugs are being used in the management of difficult behaviour (see below).

Occasionally you may be asked to help your doctor by taking the person concerned to have blood tests to check the level of a medicine in the blood (especially in the treatment of epilepsy or depression) where more accurate feedback can help to avoid unwanted side effects, determine the best dosage and understand the person's response to the treatment.

Side effects is the term usually used to describe the results of medication which are not wanted or helpful for this person. (One person's side effect may be another person's cure. For example, morphine used to control pain has the unwanted effect of causing constipation, but it is also deliberately prescribed to stop diarrhoea). Side effects may show as either an exaggerated version of what the medicine is supposed to do, such as drowsiness with a tranquilliser, or the unrelated symptom of shaking with some anti-psychotic medications. Side effects may be further complicated by drugs interacting with each other. It will be up to the doctor and pharmacist to review the effects of all the drugs an individual takes, but if there are particular concerns these should be noted so that new or different care staff can maintain a watchful eye.

Other "negative" responses to medication fall into the following categories:

• Accidental or deliberate overdose, or a build up of the drug in the body.

• Intolerance to the drug; when an individual may overreact to the usual effect of the medicine.

• Allergic reactions, such as the rash or sickness from penicillin or certain foods.

A list of the common side effects an interactions of medications being given regularly should be part of a service's "Medicine policy", particularly if the people living or working there have difficulties in alerting staff themselves about any symptoms or ill-effects.

Compliance

Compliance means "the taking of a medicine in the correct manner as prescribed" . The doctor and pharmacist should support the person with learning disabilities to make informed choices (where this is relevant, see below) and to develop a routine which enables them to continue treatment as long as necessary. Compliance can be improved by:

1. Giving clear instructions.

2. Explaining the purposes and consequences of treatment clearly.

3. Devising simplified treatment regimes

tied into other daily routines like meals or brushing teeth.

4. Treatment aids, such as the labelled foil containers which help women remember the pill.

5. Prescribing medicines which are, for the most part, safe and effective even if the person does occasionally miss a dose.

If you are aware that someone is not taking medication as prescribed, you should discuss this with the doctor so that he or she can decide on the best course of action.

Stopping medication

Serious reactions may occur if medicines are suddenly withdrawn. Again, as a member of care staff, you should not encourage service users to stop taking a medicine without discussing it with the doctor, nor should you ever decide that it would be better for the person to stop a course of tablets or a regular medicine. Any concerns you have should be discussed with the doctor or through the Individual Programme Planning meeting, but you should never make such a decision on your own.

If a team decision is taken to stop a particular drug, the doctor and carers should discuss together how best to manage the process, as some medicines give rise to specific "withdrawal" symptoms which can be distressing.

Medicine policy

Medicine policies may be used to ensure that staff are aware of the general principles of administering medicines and any particular issues which are relevant to individuals who use their service.

Medicine policies can be drawn up in collaboration between the local authority's social services department, the health authority and the Family Health Services Authority. In practice it may be put together by residential care managers and the community pharmacist and/or GP representative. Ongoing training should be carried out by the community pharmacist and other local professionals.

The policy should spell out basic principles to help staff understand and be consistent in:

• using safe procedures in handling medication

• administering medicines safely, consistently and effectively

• supporting people who are taking their own medication

• keeping accurate records of medication given so that it can be monitored and reviewed.

So policies should set out the following:

1. Training procedures in the principles of medication, the unique needs of people with learning disabilities and the legal aspects of prescribing.

2. How medicines will be stored and dosages measured out and given.

3. How medicines will be ordered and prescriptions regularly refilled.

4. When and how reviews will be held so that the effectiveness of certain medications is systematically reviewed.

5. Clarity over who should do what.

6. Instructions about record keeping of both prescribed drugs and "home remedies" and special records of symptoms or side effects to help in monitoring.

7. Instructions about when and how to help people with learning disabilities take responsibility for their own medication, which should include support and safeguards for other people living and working in the home.

Self administration

Many services aim to help people with learning disabilities to become more independent and learn new skills. People who are dependent on regular medication may need and want to take charge of their own medicines, but they will need to be actively supported and monitored in doing so, particularly if their medicine provides treatment for serious, or possibly life-threatening disorders (such as diabetes). The decision to go down this route should be taken by a number of professionals. It must be properly thought through and implemented in stages. The following factors should always be considered:

• Does the person understand and accept their need for the medicine and the effect of not taking it?

• How are they able and motivated to remember things and to manage time?

• Do they understand the instructions: when and how much of the medicine they should take, whether it should be taken before or after meals, or applied in any special way?

• What are the benefits for this person of self medication (for example they may not need to draw attention to themselves at work if they can manage their own medicine) and what are the risks (can they catch up if they miss a dose, or will it have serious consequences)?

• How will you know whether the person has taken the medication as prescribed?

Clearly there is more to such a decision than just "handing over the tablets". It is likely that you would want to start with just one dosage, maybe the person's lunchtime medication at their workplace or day centre, and then graduate to managing their medicine more completely. Care staff will have an important role in assisting this process with aids, simplified storage and availability procedures, unobtrusive random checking and reminders, and other general support.

Consent to treatment

The issue of consent is complicated and is usually determined by the individual concerned, their relatives and other relevant professionals. In the case of medical treatment it is up to the doctor to decide in the end whether the treatment they are prescribing is in that individual's "best interests". Thus although you may be consulted about whether you think someone understands a decision, you should not take it on yourself to avoid medical treatment or referral because the person "does not like doctors" or is "choosing" not to keep a hospital appointment.

On the whole people with severe learning disabilities are deemed not to be able to give their consent, and although no one else is legally empowered to do so on their behalf, a doctor would usually prescribe the same treatment which they and their colleagues would prescribe for someone with the same condition who did not have a learning disability. Obviously the more serious and complex the condition the more likely it is that a "professional" decision would be made on the person's behalf (see table below).

Services should have a formalised process for consulting and making decisions in this area. Changing circumstances may affect individuals who have additional mental health or behavioural problems, and ethical issues are particularly relevant when prescribing contraceptives or sexually suppressant medications. Some treatments or operations such as abortion or sterilisation are usually referred to court to ensure that the pros and cons are carefully considered. The law in this area is currently under review.

Special medical needs

People with learning disabilities tend to need *more* medical treatment than the general population. Common conditions include neurological, eye, skin, mental health and orthopaedic problems. In general the more severe the learning disability, the greater the medical problems.

Older age
On the whole the medical needs of elderly people with a mild degree of learning disability are no different from those of the general population. There may however be specific associations between the cause of learning disabilities and the ageing process – for example people with Down's Syndrome are at risk of developing Alzheimer's Disease (dementia), hearing and visual impairments and thyroid disorders.

Common mental health problems in elderly people include dementia, depression, psychotic symptoms, confusion and anxiety. It is important that Alzheimer's Disease be considered in any middle-aged person with Down's Syndrome who has developed behaviour problems, or loss of memory, intellectual functions or social skills.

The ageing process in the body may result in the need for smaller doses of medication and a greater likelihood of side effects.

Epilepsy
Epilepsy is a common additional handicap for people with a learning disability. The clinical presentation depends on the location of abnormal nerve cells and the

frequency of excessive electrical discharges. Fits or seizures may further damage intellectual functioning; temporal lobe epilepsy has associations with psychosis and depression; and the social effects of the condition have an impact on psychological wellbeing.

Certain anti-epileptic medications may cause or exacerbate behaviour problems. Other side-effects can include slurred speech, poor coordination, overgrowth of gums, coarsening of facial features and changes in body hair – with obvious effects on the person's self-esteem.

Mental health

People with learning disabilities have also been shown to be at greater risk of developing mental illness or behaviour disorders. This is likely to be a consequence of many factors, including:
• epilepsy
• brain damage
• health problems
• the use of medications
• special sensory problems
• communication difficulties
• an increased number of negative or stressful life events.

The diagnosis of mental health problems in people with learning disabilities is often difficult, as there may be problems of communication and the symptoms may not be typical, so look for and report any change in the person's usual behaviour rather than any specific symptoms.

The important disorders when considering the use of medication are the psychotic and depressive illnesses. Care staff must be particularly aware of the purpose, use and side effects of anti-psychotic medications and anti-depressants. People with learning disabilities may have increased brain sensitivity and susceptibility to side effects.

Medical treatment of behaviour disorders

Sometimes anti-psychotic medications, or other drugs, are given in treatment of behaviour disorders or self-injury. The theory of use is based on the tranquillising effect and the reduction in the person's level of arousal. It must be emphasised that these drugs are best used in the short term, and should not be considered in isolation from other interventions – social, environmental, psychological, behavioural and educational (see Chapter 7 on Challenging Behaviour). Medical treatment is likely to be more successful if there is an underlying health problem.

Conclusion

Maintaining good health for people with learning disabilities requires consistent cooperation between care staff, the patient and their doctor. You do not need to be a medical expert to act sensibly on the person's behalf, just willing to maintain and pass on information and records so that the doctor can make the best decisions about treatment, and do your best to see that treatment is carried out.

Points to remember

1. Follow the doctor's instructions about taking medicines, exactly and consistently.
2. Don't suddenly stop regular medication without proper consultation.
3. Store medicines carefully and keep records of both prescribed medication and "home remedies".
4. Be familiar with the purpose of medicines prescribed and their side effects.
5. Encourage the development of a comprehensive medicine policy that is relevant to the needs of people with learning disabilties and care staff.
6. Encourage self-medication only with proper planning and support.
7. Good health relies on collaboration between care staff, GPs and other health professionals.

CHAPTER 19

Rights, advocacy and support

Kathy West

• Human rights we all share: how to claim and defend them for people with learning disabilities • Self-advocacy and assertiveness training • Citizen advocacy • Legal advice and representation • Complaints • Giving support

This chapter is about the rights which people with learning difficulties have under the law. It is also about some of the ways those rights can be claimed and defended, either through their own efforts, or with the help and support of others.

On the whole, adult people with learning disabilities have the same rights and protections under the law as anyone. The United Nations International Declaration of Human Rights, which has been adopted by member nations, places a moral obligation on those nations to respect human rights and makes no exceptions for people who have disabilities. It proclaims the equal rights of all people to human dignity and freedom.

Another declaration, that of the International League of societies which act on behalf of people with learning disabilities, was signed by participating organisations in many nations and applied these broad human rights more specifically to the particular needs of people with learning disabilities.

The "Declaration of General and Special Rights of the Mentally Retarded"[1] included the principles above, which although they have no force in

> **People with learning disabilities have the same basic rights as other citizens of the same country and same age:**
> • the right to proper medical care, education and training
> • the right to economic security and a decent standard of living
> • the right to live with their own family
> • the right to leisure activities
> • the right to live in as normal circumstances as possible
> • the right to protection from exploitation, abuse and degrading treatment, and proper legal safeguards
> • above all the right to respect.

international law, stated the aims of international societies.

Thus both UK laws and world declarations of human rights support the view that all people, whatever their race, sex, disability, colour, class, or national origin should be entitled to equal rights, opportunities, dignity and respect. The reality is often unfortunately far short of this, particularly when people are at a disadvantage because of disability. So it is especially important that people with disabilities and those who work with them, learn about their rights.

Rights in practice

Having rights is one thing; being able to use them is another. The aim of **advocacy** in all its forms is to ensure that people with learning disabilities are not deprived of their rights through lack of information, lack of resources, lack of someone to speak up for them, or through active abuse or exploitation.

There are many different kinds of advocacy. A dictionary definition says that advocacy is "active support" and an advocate is "a person who upholds or defends a cause; a supporter or a person who pleads his/her client's cause in a court of law". In the informal sense, we are all likely to call on other people, especially friends or family, if we have a problem or are in need of advice. Sometimes we ask other people for their active help.

And from time to time, in a more formal sense, we may call on the services of a lawyer, or a Citizen's Advice Bureau, or someone to help to figure out benefits or help with consumer problems. We may also speak up for ourselves when facing problems, or join together with others who have a similar problem or issue to face, in self help groups.

Advocacy for people with learning disabilities takes all of these forms, and it is especially important that they are available, when for many speaking up is a very difficult thing to do.

Self advocacy

Self advocacy is about people speaking for themselves, either as individuals or through a group. People with learning difficulties, who often have difficulties speaking, have a surprising amount to say, especially if there are good listeners to hear, a safe place to say things, and plenty of time and encouragement.

Self advocacy is possible in many ways. It ranges from supporting individuals to speak and give their opinions at meetings, to encouraging groups of people to form their own views and enabling the development of independent groups, run by people themselves, but perhaps supported by others.

In the long term the most important kind of self advocacy is independent self advocacy. This happens in organisations such as People First, where groups of people with learning disabilities get together, usually with the support of one or more advisers, and are independent of any services.

There are also other independent self advocacy groups in the UK which operate in local areas - these may be part of an area advocacy group run by people with disabilities, a tenant's association run by tenants of community based housing schemes, or special interest and activity groups.

People first

People First is the best known of the independent self-advocacy groups for people with learning disabilities. The original groups started in the 1970s in the USA, and there are now hundreds of groups in many different countries. Every two or three years People First holds an international conference, where people with learning disabilities and their advisers and supporters get together from all over the world.

The name People First is a statement by members that they are human beings first and that their disabilities are second. They want to be seen as people who have value and dignity and an important role to play in the community.

There are other kinds of self advocacy groups which help to encourage people to learn new ways of speaking up and join with others to pursue interests and make their views known. "Speak for yourself" or Self-Advocacy groups are becoming quite common in Adult Education Institutes, Day Centres and residential settings.

This is how the People First group in the state of Washington (USA) explains the importance of self-advocacy[2]:

> **Why we need self-advocacy and self-help groups like People First**
>
> In the past, and even today, adults with disabilities are:
> • treated like children
> • not given a chance to speak up and participate in decisions about their lives
> • labelled and called names
> • locked up in institutions
> • not told about their rights and responsibilities as citizens
> • not given a chance to show that they can live, work, participate and contribute to the community
> • not given many choices about their lives
> • not seen as valuable people and given the respect and dignity they deserve as human beings.

What do self-advocacy groups do?

– Meet regularly and encourage each other to participate;
– support each other and solve problems
– learn new skills, such as how to run meetings;
– do things together – outings, parties, sports, films, etc;
– raise funds;
– publish a newsletter;
– learn about rights;
– help build each other's confidence and learn to act assertively;
– make their views known - to the Council, to MPs, to managers of services;
– find new members;
– send speakers to other groups and organise local conferences;

– have fun;
– take action: write letters, hold a public meeting, go on a march, visit the local MP.

Advice and support

Groups like People First do need support from advisers, especially in the early days. It often takes two or three years for a group to get going, learn the skills of running meetings and what the officers do, and gain confidence to take on most of the work. An adviser needs to be an equal partner, but must take a lead from the group, rather than directing the group in the way they think best. They need to be a good listener, to check out actions and feelings with members, and to ensure that their actions help to increase members' feelings of self-confidence and independence.

There are many kinds of support which advisers and supporters can offer that can be helpful to people wanting to speak for themselves:

– just being there; offering a word of encouragement and a friendly smile
– helping to boost someone's confidence by taking notice of their efforts and achievements; being on their side
– encouraging people to try new skills, perhaps as one small step at a time; being enthusiastic about progress
– using different ways to communicate and learn people's wishes and interests, especially when they find speech difficult or impossible
– offering practical help and support
– working actively towards greater independence.

Assertiveness training

Many self-advocacy groups, self-defence groups and social skills groups learn to act more assertively. Some of the things taught include:

• how to say no;

• how to ask for time to think about something;

• asking why;

• how to start a conversation;

• learning what your rights are;

• how to ask for what you want in a firm and polite way;

• speaking and looking more confident;

• saying what you're feeling and thinking, rather than expecting people to read your mind;

• learning how to make your point and ensure people listen to you.

Individual self advocacy can also take place in many ways when people with learning disabilities are encouraged to have a say and what they say is listened to. It might mean holding a conference or consultation where people are asked to come along and say what they think. It might mean that when services are evaluated special efforts are made to ask people what they think of them, and these answers are fed back into the planning process. It certainly means that when there are reviews or planning meetings about individuals, they are fully included in the process, given support to speak up, and their preferences and wishes are recorded and acted upon. This will ideally include someone of their own choice to help represent their views and offer support (see Chapter 4 on Individual Planning).

Citizen advocacy

Citizen advocacy[3] is a particular form of advocacy which first began to develop quite widely in North America in the 1970s. It was seen as a way of involving ordinary citizens in the community with other people who were at a disadvantage – because of a learning disability, physical disability, mental illness, homelessness, being from an ethnic minority, or for other reasons.

Ordinary people have many skills they can share with others and many links with friends and activities in their local community. As they would not be employees of service providers they might be able to maintain a longer relationship, and it was hoped that they would be more committed as they would not be paid to offer support.

Citizen advocates were seen as needing particular qualities, which required that they were more than just a friend who might share time and activities. In this country there are a growing number of citizen advocacy schemes, as well as other befriending and volunteer schemes which do some of the same things.

A citizen advocate is someone who

• agrees to enter into a long term relationship. It takes time to get to know a person well and to build up trust. It is usually over time that having a good friend makes a real difference to someone's life.

• does not work for a major service provider to the person, in order to prevent conflicts of interest. The advocate can't be a staff member involved with the person.

• is unpaid. They are in the relationship because they want to be rather than because they are paid to be there.

• has minimum conflicts of interest so that the loyalty is to the person with learning disabilities and not for example, to an employer or the person's wider family. Thus they can truly represent the person's own points of view.

• will respect a person's rights, viewpoints and wishes and be committed to confidentiality about personal matters.

Many staff members see themselves as advocates, and indeed they can have an

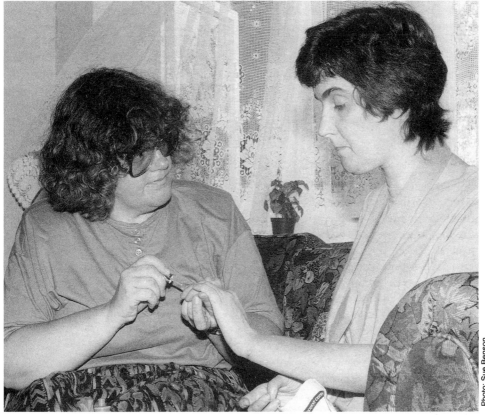

Just being with someone, showing your interest and commitment – in this case while applying the nail varnish she enjoys wearing – is very important. It can take a lot of time to build up trust.

important role to play promoting people's interests. However, this role is necessarily limited, because staff are not independent. Often staff have to take a group's interests into account rather than those of specific individuals, or policies won't allow them to speak out, or they risk being disciplined by their employers. Often staff turnover is high, and resources and relationships with other staff members may affect what is possible.

Thus, independent advocacy is very important. It can feel a bit scary for a staff team to open up their service in this way but in the long run it makes things more interesting and provides a safety net and a spur to good practice.

Other kinds of advocacy: Self advocacy and citizen advocacy are especially important. But we should not overlook the more ordinary kinds of support available to all members of the community.

Citizens' Advice Bureaux

Citizen's Advice Bureaux (CABs), Consumer Advice Centres, Benefits and Housing Advice Centres, Community Health Councils, and so on.

These should be available to members of the community who have learning disabilities in the same way as to anyone else – for advice, representation, help with making complaints, and the like. It is true that many are not used to being approached by people with learning disabilities, so we need to encourage this.

Sometimes an approach by members of

a self-advocacy group, a citizen advocate, or a staff member can help to smooth the way and get an advice centre to think how they could be more welcoming and more supportive. It may require a longer campaign to persuade ordinary advice centres that they have a role in supporting people with learning disabilities.

Legal advice

Legal advice and representation should also be available for people with learning disabilities. As most people in this group are poor, they are likely to be eligible for legal aid. A frequent issue is when people have little or no communication, and can not be said to be giving informed consent to action being taken on their behalf.

As most lawyers are not used to dealing with people with learning difficulties, there is often a place for a person's own representative – such as a keyworker – to pave the way or even offer support throughout. This is especially true when the person needing legal representation has little or no ordinary speech.

Sometimes when a person needs to have legal action taken on their behalf, but it is judged by a doctor that they are incapable of giving consent, then the Solicitor General can agree that a solicitor can take action on their behalf – this might be, for example, where they have been injured in an accident through negligence, and they would benefit from receiving compensation for their injuries, or if they are about to have a major operation such as a sterilisation or abortion.

Complaints to social services

Since April 1991 all social services departments have been required under community care legislation to operate complaints procedures relating to anything to do with social services.

Complaints can be made, for example, about lack of services, changes in or refusals of services, the ways in which they are delivered (quality of service) or the way a service user has been dealt with.

People with learning difficulties should be encouraged to complain and offered support to do so if necessary. If people cannot complain themselves, someone – an advocate, family member, friend – can do so on their behalf.

In one local authority area, for example, people with learning difficulties have complained about:

• a proposal to withdraw their weekly day centre payments;

• being repeatedly hit by someone living in the same house;

• transport being repeatedly late;

• having adult education classes cut;

• the loss of a mini-bus.

Many people with learning difficulties do not have enough speech or writing skills or confidence to manage everything by themselves. Often a part of the problem is that they are frightened – of being hurt, or losing services or of being victimised. This is when an outside supporter can provide special help, and in some cases take up an issue on someone else's behalf.

Support can be given in many ways: for example, by using someone's own words and putting them into a letter; accompanying someone when they make their complaint to give them confidence; looking for the ways in which the problem affects the person and making a complaint on their behalf.

Other ways to complain

Any local person can complain or make their views known in a variety of other ways. Local advice centres can often suggest the best way. it might mean approaching local councillors, MPs, the local government ombudsman, the customer relations manager in a local firm, and so forth. Many people will need help and support to do this, and in many places local organisations will provide a representative, supporter or advocate to help out.

Under the Disabled Person's Act 1986, all people with disabilities should have been able either to appoint their own representatives to take up issues on their behalf or be able to have a representative if they couldn't choose one themselves. While this part of the Act has never been brought into force, good practice now promotes the possibility of many more people having their own representatives or advocates to make sure their views and needs are known at meetings about the services which are offered to them.

How to help

There are many ways in which advocates, advocacy supporters and staff members can help people with learning disabilities to speak for themselves and find ways of expressing their wishes and viewpoints. Some have already been mentioned. Here are a few more ideas:

• Helping people to find new and better ways to communicate (see Chapter 5)

• For people who don't talk, keeping records or a diary of when someone is happy, alert, shows interest or is anxious, angry or distressed, can be very helpful. Such a record is useful to look at over time and give clues to someone's progress, preferences, feelings and interests. The information can be contributed to making plans for individuals.

• Using photographs, films and videos can be helpful. People are often enthusiastic about things but cannot talk about them. There are also many films and videos which have been made by and for people with learning disabilities. Home videos or audio tapes including the person him or herself can provoke some enthusiastic responses and give many clues to what a person likes.[4]

• Paying attention to a person's first language and culture is very important. Many people who come from families where a language other than English is spoken often know and understand words in this language, and should get support to develop and use this knowledge. Foods, customs, pictures, music and other links with the person's confidence and helping them to feel good about themselves. Advocates who are of a person's own race or culture can provide valuable support, because people from minority ethnic backgrounds face double discrimination (see Chapter 13).

• Using music, and getting people involved in art, music and other creative activities can be a way to communicate. One young woman in South London is a marvellous artist, and can draw and paint many beautiful and recognisable things, but she has no speech or sign language.

• Patience is vital. it sometimes takes weeks or months for changes and developments to happen, but these are often even more worthwhile when they do happen. Many self-advocacy groups take over three years before becoming strong enough to be independent. It takes lots of time to learn how to listen, to take turns speaking, to run a meeting, to gain confidence. Individuals with severe disabilities may take months just to recognise someone.

• Just being with someone can be very important - a way of showing your interest and commitment. Sometimes it takes a lot of time for trust to build up, and many people with learning disabilities have been let down countless times by other people. After a while, just being with someone and paying attention (even if not talking), a person will begin to get the idea that you are there for them.

• People with learning disabilities should have the same rights as anyone else to dignity, respect, privacy, services, protection under the law, and so forth. So often this is not what they experience. So it is worth any advocate or supporter or staff member asking themselves regularly: "Is what I am observing in Mr X's or Ms Y's life what I would like or expect for myself?" If the answer is no, then it is time for some action or support.

Points to remember

1. People with learning disabilities have the same rights under the law as everyone else, with very few exceptions.

2. They are also entitled to the same human rights as anyone else – above all respect.

3. It is important that as many people as possible know their own rights and how to claim them.

4. Self-advocacy opportunities give people a chance to speak and communicate for themselves.

5. It is also important to have advocates who can help to represent the views of individuals with learning disabilities. An independent viewpoint is important.

6. Support for people can be vital in order to help them communicate their own viewpoint: to boost confidence, provide

them with expert advice and help with communication difficulties.

References

1. The International League of Societies for the Mentally Handicapped, 1968.

2. People First Leadership Training Manual, National People First Project, 1988, Downsview, Ontario, Canada.

3. For more information about Citizen Advocacy contact National Citizen Advocacy, Unit K, Leroy House, 436 Essex Road, London N1 3OP. Tel: 071 359 8289.

4. People First has a list of materials for self-advocacy groups and advisers, which include books, pamphlets, tapes and videos. It can be obtained by contacting: People First, Instrument House, 207-215 Kings Cross Road, London WC1X 9DB. Tel: 071 713 6400.

Useful books

Alcoe J and Brown H (1989). *Five Star Group Work* - a group work manual for service users. Pavilion Publishing, (Brighton) Ltd, 42 Lansdowne Place, Hove, East Sussex BN3 1HH.
Crawley, Bronach, and others (1988). *Learning About Self-Advocacy* (Booklets 1-5), CHM, London. Available from Values into Action, Oxford House, Derbyshire Street, London E2 6HG.
Whittaker, Andrea (1991). *Supporting Self-Advocacy*, Kings Fund Centre, 126 Albert Street, London NW1 7NF. Tel: 071 267 6112.
Worrell, Bill (1988). *People First Advice for Advisors*, National People First Project, Ontario, Canada. Available from People First in London (address above).

CHAPTER 20
How the home is managed

Jayne Kilgallen

• How care staff are selected • How you and your manager relate to each other • Training and supervision • Your responsibilities

Like all homes, residential services need to be well-managed. As you know from your own home experiences, this is by no means an easy task. Some days when people are ill or short of money there is certainly "no place like home".

This chapter identifies the key areas for care staff in understanding what managing the home entails. It should make clear to you what your responsibilities are as a case assistant, how your job fits in to the management structure, and how you and your manager should relate to each other. It should also help you if you have to "act up" during your manager's absence, or if you are aiming to be a manager yourself in the future.

Selecting staff

One of the manager's main jobs is appointing staff. Care staff are recruited from a wide variety of backgrounds: some of you may have had previous work or voluntary experience with people with learning difficulties, but for some of you this will be a completely new experience.

The manager starts with a "person specification", containing the criteria by which candidates are appointed. Each application is checked against this person specification, for shortlisting before some are asked to come for interview.

CARE STAFF: PERSON SPECIFICATION

Essential:

1. A positive attitude towards supporting people with learning difficulties to lead as full a life as possible in the local community.

2. Ability to work on own initiative, to encourage and support people with learning disabilities to take up a range of activities in the community.

3. Willingness and ability to develop new skills and to respond to new ideas flexibly.

4. Basic literacy skills: ability to complete entries in clients' records on activities and events, ability to read and understand service policies.

5. Basic numeracy: ability to monitor clients' personal spending and maintain a balance in records of expenditure.

Desirable:

1. Previous experience of working with people with learning difficulties.

2. Previous experience of working in a team.

The whole recruitment and selection programme should take place within an equal opportunities framework which ensures that no candidate is discriminated against for reasons of ethnic origin, age, gender or sexual orientation.

During your interview you should be given information about the type of people you will be working with. It is important that you ask about this and check out anything you are not sure about. Don't be afraid that people will think you silly – it's their job to give you as much information as possible.

And so to work

Starting any new job is for all of us a difficult time. All those new people to get to know and new tasks when all around you appear to know exactly what they're doing. Your manager will understand your feelings and ensure you get additional support during those first days.

However, from time to time some care staff take up post only to find that they are not happy. If this happens to you it is vital that you discuss your feelings will your line manager; they will help you to sort out what it is that's making you unhappy and discuss options to assist you. For some people however the situation may not be so easily resolved and re-deployment or in extreme cases alternative employment may be the only option.

Do remember though that most people at some stage or other have doubts about their chosen career. With the right support and perseverance most continue with their job and develop their career.

Management structures

What's a line manager? This is your "boss" - the person who supports and nurtures you (and occasionally tells you off)!

Each service will have its own clearly laid out management structure which may be like this:

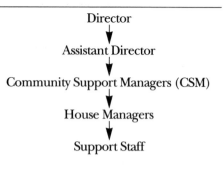

Ask your manager to tell you where your unit fits in, and find out how many other services your agency runs.

Supervision

Supervision is a one to one meeting – you with your line manager. All staff of all levels should receive supervision. A session might last between one and two hours and is conducted in a quiet private space. This is your opportunity to discuss work related issues with your line manager, and they will give you feedback on your performance.

It is not a session to "catch you out" or "tell you off", it is about you and your work and will enable you to develop your skills, set objectives and identify your training needs. Sometimes a "supervision contract" is worked out, which states clearly who is doing what.

You may also receive supervision "on the job" more informally when your line manager works alongside you. During this time they will give you practical advice about supporting particular people with learning disabilities, and will guide you and enable you to work more effectively by showing you what to do. This will also provide an opportunity for them to give you helpful and positive feedback on your performance.

It is important that you do receive supervision. If you don't, or feel that it's too infrequent, discuss this with your line manager.

Training

Much of your training will be given on the job by your line manager and on occasions other managers. However, it is likely that you'll receive an initial induction training. This may be spread over a fortnight and should provide you with the basic skills and knowledge you need for the job. It should cover such things as:

• Service philosophies
• Role of care staff
• Epilepsy, first aid, hepatitis B
• Skills teaching
• Lifting and handling
• Sexuality and personal relationships
• Challenging behaviour
• Policies and procedures (eg finance, medication)
• Individual planning

As you continue your career other courses will be available (see Chapter 22).

Accountability

The job of care staff is, to say the least, extremely varied - "a Jack of all Trades". To make life even more complicated this is set within a framework of policies, procedures and boundaries for staff. These provide the "rules" within which you have to do your job and make everyday decisions.

The major areas that you will be responsible for are:

Finance: Each person will be receiving benefits and have personal money that they have to budget for. Many people with learning disabilities will always need support in this area, while others will gain some independence. To protect people with learning disabilities from financial abuse and to ensure that their rights to receive and be actively involved in accounting for their money are protected, each service should have developed a clearly defined policy and procedures. It is essential that this is followed as it also acts as a protection for staff against allegations of stealing.

If you are worried about any aspect of this, talk to your line manager.

Part of your work will involve your supporting people in social and leisure activities such as swimming, going to the pub or cinema. The service will provide money to pay for you to do this; you should not be out of pocket. Each service's procedure for doing this varies – so find out.

Reporting of incidents: An "incident" is when something unusual occurs which involves injury or distress to people. It may be an incident of aggression towards another person with learning disabilities, or an accident in which someone is injured.

It is your responsibility to note the incident and write all the details down on an incident form. If the incident is serious in nature and you need advice, contact your line manager in office hours or whoever is on call outside office hours.

Administering medicine: For safety and legal reasons all medication must be kept in a lockable cupboard and administered according to strict procedures.

You will receive training on this procedure and you will be instructed as to how to administer and record medicines given (see chapter 18).

Confidentiality

A part of your work will involve receiving confidential information about the people with learning disabilities you are working with. This means you are entrusted with information which you are expected to respect. Communicating confidential information to outside bodies without authority will be regarded by the service as a very serious matter.

Care staff should therefore be aware of guidelines regarding handling of confidential information. If you are in any doubt contact your line manager. On other occasions you are required *not* to keep things confidential: for example, if you are told someone may be being mistreated or abused.

Being a role model

One of the major aspects of your job as a member of the care staff is to act as a role model for the people with learning disabilities you work with.

What does this mean? Well, it means that your behaviour around the house gives them messages about normal social behaviour, what is acceptable and what isn't. Always be aware of this and think how you will be perceived by others. People with learning disabilities look to you for a lead.

Part of your job will involve you being in the community with people with learning disabilities. You will be a key person in helping them to make contact with members of the public. This often means trying harder; being diplomatic and trying to work around any prejudice you encounter; sometimes biting your tongue (without apologising for the person's learning difficulty).

In practice it means taking your empty glasses back to the bar on leaving and saying thank you; it means ensuring you leave no mess; it means not reacting to the general public's stares and glares; in short it means being on your "best behaviour". Many times a well-meaning, well-intentioned care staff member has argued too strongly or abruptly and too loudly, for all the right reasons but in the end putting people off.

Consistency

Consistency is a necessary component of any staff team. It is important that all team members use the same approach with people with learning disabilities. On occasions you may disagree with the approach that has been agreed. Although you will get a chance to air your disagreement you will be expected to stick to any agreed plans; to "give it a go". These will then be reviewed and discussed with the whole staff team, and amendments made in the light of experience. This is especially important when working with people who have difficult behaviours (see chapter 7).

Team meetings

As a member of a team you will probably have regular team meetings (approximately every three weeks). These will normally be chaired by the house manager, and minutes will be taken, written up and circulated. On occasions other people may be invited, for example senior managers or members of the Community Mental Handicap Team.

Before the meeting an agenda will be drawn up, so if you have something you want to raise you should put it on the agenda:

TYPICAL TEAM MEETING AGENDA
1. Service user issues - activities people have been involved in this week:
• update on recent hospital appointment for Robert • how to deal with John when he scratches Amanda
2. House issues:
• new shower • ordering new curtains
• next month's rota
3. Training – session on how to respond if Jane has an epileptic fit
4. Any other business.

CHAPTER 21

How to manage an emergency

Heather Hughes

• Emergencies can and should be planned for • Factors that can make an emergency more likely, and how to avoid them • How to consult and make your plans as a team • Medical emergencies • Challenging behaviour

Almost everyone is called upon to deal with an emergency at some time in their lives. In my life, emergencies have included running out of petrol in a strange place without any money, and having to put out a chip pan fire following my brother's first attempt to cook his own meal (sexist? but true!).

Almost all emergencies are avoidable. Many everyday "emergencies" could have been anticipated; they most frequently involve forgetting about or forgetting to do something.

In this chapter, we are going to look at how to "predict" emergencies and how to respond to them. Many emergency or crisis situations build up over a period of time, which means you have some time to plan and sometimes even avert the emergency. With a little forward planning and thought, most emergency situations come to seem more predictable and therefore less uncontrollable.

Planning ahead

We expect our emergency services, the police, fire and ambulance brigades, to know what to do when we ring them. We expect that they have had experience of the same kind of situations before and have worked out the answers or, at least, can implement some procedures which are likely to work.

This competence from our emergency services has not come about by chance. It is the result of training, practice, learning from mistakes and changing or amending procedures. The same is true of working in human services. Someone going missing, forgetting to go shopping, somebody cutting themselves on a knife or becoming seriously ill, are all "emergencies" which have happened time and time again. Good services however have worked out ways of responding, procedures which make the emergency less panicky.

Some services work in the belief that when you work with people with learning disabilities, you must experience more emergencies than is usual. I do not think this is true. What it reflects is that we often do not plan well enough to support people with additional needs.

The idea of planning beforehand may seem a strange one. But actually very few crises are unique: there are usually people around who have experienced similar situations to the one you might find yourself in. It should not be too difficult to use their experiences to help you plan. Start from the following golden rules:

• Have a general plan setting out how you will react or what you will do, ready and easily available.

• Don't panic; stay calm whatever happens – however hard that might be.

• Get help, preferably alerting someone before you need it. Don't try to cope on your own.

It is important to remember that some crises or emergencies are not over and done with in a few minutes. There is a range of possible lengths of time for emergencies: quick moments of challenging behaviour; medium term emergencies such as accompanying someone to the accident and emergency department of the hospital or looking for someone who has left the house; and longer term emergencies such as ongoing shortage of staff due to illness.

Managing emergencies

Most emergencies and crises have beginnings, middles and ends: they do not spring from nowhere. There are four quite separate stages to the development of an emergency:

• The skills and ability of staff and management to "cope with" and manage it;

• the build up to the emergency, and things which contribute to it – "fuel to the fire";

• the emergency or crisis itself and how it is managed;

• "mopping up" and debriefing afterwards.

Every time you experience an emergency or a "near miss" you ought to talk through each of these four stages with your colleagues and managers. The focus of the discussion should be to think about what could be done differently next time which would allow you to avert the crisis or lessen its intensity and effects. Thus you can use the framework above to develop your own crisis or emergency management plans and procedures. The sign of a good service is not the number of emergencies it survives, but how many it avoids!

Staff skills: can you cope?

Many crises in services are only a surprise because there is a lack of, or inadequate, monitoring. There are a number of signals which will directly or indirectly indicate if a service is likely to be approaching a crisis. Some that I keep a watch on are:

• Is there a chronic staff shortage?

• How often are there staff changes in that team?

• How "difficult" is the group of people with learning disabilities – for example in terms of their behaviour, the extent to which they can communicate with you, and whether they have a lot of physical disabilities?

• How much training do the staff get, especially in the work setting?

• How much time do the managers of the service spend there, and how much do they know about the needs of the people being cared for?

• Do the staff get regular supervision and appraisal, and if so, what is the quality of their service?

You can add ideas from your own experience about what other factors could be monitored.

Whether you will experience a crisis is not usually down to just one thing but a mixture of different things. For example, a service may be able to support being understaffed, but not when its manager goes off on long term sick leave and someone's difficult behaviour gets worse. If the items which I have included on the list above are working well, they make the service more capable of supporting the needs of both staff and people with learning disabilities.

The build up

When something serious happens in life, and everyone has calmed down afterwards it is easy to look back with "the benefit of hindsight". That is to say we can see that all the signs were there if only we hadn't been too busy, too involved or too disinterested to see them. The same is true in services, and is particularly common when everyone's attention is focused on one aspect of a situation and not on the other things which might well be quietly developing into crises and emergencies of their own.

For example, the death of a service user may result in staff and management talking about that person all the time, partly because *they* need to and partly because there are a lot of arrangements to be made. A possible knock-on effect of this on other service users is that they may well feel less valued than the person who has died, or start worrying about their own death. They may never really have liked the person who died very much anyway, and object to being included in the bereavement of others.

This kind of scenario can result in people taking extreme courses of action, such as not eating, or losing their tempers. This may exacerbate what is already a difficult situation, into an emergency or even a crisis.

Get help before you need it

In the section on getting additional help, you will get some ideas about who to call on for what. The important thing to remember at this point is to call for help *before* you need it. The help you need might take a variety of forms, depending on the kind of crisis.

• If you are in any doubt about whether what is happening could result in an emergency or crisis, ring a service manager and talk it over. This will clarify the situation for you, and alert the manager that help might be needed soon.

• If managers do not respond to this approach, or if the potential for crisis is building up over time, put your anxieties and queries in writing and discuss them at supervision or at the next team meeting.

• If you continue to get an unsatisfactory response, possibly because you are the only person who can see the potential for crisis, put it in writing to your manager and send a copy of your letter to their manager. This will rarely be ignored, but if it is, and a crisis does develop, at least you can say "I told you so". I am sure that several memos were sent predicting the Chernobyl disaster, for example – it is not only care services that ignore their staff!

Remember you are the person who will be left to manage the emergency and possibly protect yourself, other staff and other people with learning disabilities. Your organisation has a responsibility to reassure you that all these people will be safe, physically and emotionally.

The emergency itself

In many ways, this is the easy bit! What I mean by that is that either you know what to do or you don't. If you do, then you'll get on with it calmly and efficiently. If you don't, then you'll either panic and be no good to anybody and possibly make the whole thing worse, or you'll do the best you can in a very difficult situation, drawing on your knowledge and expertise from similar situations, and possibly things you have read or seen on TV.

Later in this chapter, you will find some more detailed advice on getting additional help. You are likely to need to call for additional help in an emergency, whether it is to find someone who knows the "missing persons" policy off by heart, to update a manager about someone's behaviour or feelings at that time, or just to seek reassurance that you are doing the right thing.

I have found it useful to keep a list of all potential sources of help and their phone numbers near to every phone in the house. You never know how quickly you might need to dial. This has saved me valuable minutes in a crisis and served me well on one occasion when it was the phone in the staff sleeping room which got damaged. Scrabbling around trying to find the number of the person's GP, or the psychiatric emergency clinic, is not a recommended procedure for helping you stay calm. Again, being able to direct another person to the address book saying "Phone Dr Jones - the number is under D for doctor" also helps you keep calm, gives the other person something to do and reassures them that you are in control.

Debriefing

This is the worst bit, in my experience, because it is often badly attended to. There are two stages to the debriefing: immediately afterwards and some time afterwards.

Immediately afterwards, what you're often left with is loads of adrenalin pumping around your system which you don't really need any more but you don't know what to do with. Everybody asks you how you are and tells you that you did a great job (even when you didn't). You might go out and "party" afterwards or you might burst into tears of relief, or you might feel really angry at yourself, at the person who caused or was the subject of the emergency, or at nobody in particular. You might be given the opportunity to go to a quiet place and have a cup of tea while you fill out an incident report.

Think about the last emergency or crisis you were involved in. What helped you get over it? Talking to somebody; going for a swim; doing something practical; being on your own for ten minutes; what? Work with your team in team meetings and get them to identify what makes them feel better in that situation. Write it down and you've got the first part of your individualised debriefing strategy.

The next stage ought to be for your manager to talk through exactly what happened with you – a formal "debriefing". This might happen one hour, or a day later, depending on the situation or the individual. The aims of debriefing ought to be both to make you feel better about what happened and also to modify existing service procedures. Unfortunately however, the experience of most people I talk to seems to be that it either doesn't happen at all, in the spirit of "least said, soonest mended", or is done only if there is the possibility of somebody, somewhere being disciplined.

People usually need to talk about what has happened to them, particularly if it has been stressful. Where people have not been debriefed properly by someone within the service, then they will work to find somebody else to talk to, possibly somebody inappropriate, risking damage to a reputation, usually either that of the person with learning disabilities involved, or the manager. Sometimes both will be damaged and confidentiality broken. Additionally, and by no means least, the feelings and emotions of the staff involved will never be resolved and put to rest. This can itself make an emergency or crisis more likely to happen in the future.

Talk to your manager about how he or she would debrief staff following different kinds of emergency. Get the staff team to talk about how they think different incidents *should* be debriefed. What are the similarities and differences? Are there situations which seem to need to be debriefed in the same way?

Some items which you might find on a checklist of positive responses are:

• Remove any remaining immediate risk of crisis. Organise bank/agency cover if required.

• Talk to staff involved in the incident as soon as possible – preferably in person but by phone if necessary – to check out the situation and their immediate feelings. Organise bank/agency cover if required.

• Arrange the time, venue and people for an immediate (or within 24 hours) debrief.

• At this time, confirm with service staff the "official story" of this incident. Check back through incident reports involving previous behaviour or events like this.

• Read the incident report from this event together.

• Interviews with staff involved should include asking them about:
– how they are feeling
– the build up to the crisis, including their response
– the crisis itself and what happened
– what happened and how they felt immediately after the crisis.

– how they feel about returning to work:

Do they need a manager or another named person to go back with them till they rebuild their confidence?

Do they need additional time off, or not to work a "sleep over" shift (for example)

for a few days until they have completely recovered?

Is there any immediate training we can deliver which would relieve the situation now and/or in the future?

• Decide on a date to check out how everyone is later.

• Write up the interviews, attach to the incident sheet and put a copy in the file of the staff members concerned and the person with learning disabilities involved.

• Discuss the incident and its possible relationship with similar events in the service, at the managers' meeting.

• Make any appropriate changes to service responses and procedures.

Some situations have been so stressful, or have gone on for such a long time, that some additional debriefing or even counselling might be required.

Getting additional help

Finding out which other people or agencies can help you is often the first thing to know in preparing to face emergencies. When you call them, and in what circumstances, should be specified in advance. In difficult or stressful situations, it is easy to overreact and ask for help from everybody you can find. This "sweeping" movement is usually unhelpful and can damage reputations – both yours and that of the person with learning disabilities. However, this statement needs to be balanced against the requirement to ask for help or alert support services before you need them. Knowing that help is nearby or on its way might also give you the confidence you need to manage and avert an emergency.

Management on call
Most services have a management "on call" system which is available to offer

additional support in unusual or stressful circumstances. Is there such a system in your organisation? Do you know who to call and for what kinds of things? More importantly perhaps, would they know what to do if you called them?

Get together a list of things that have happened to you at work which you think have been real emergencies or "near misses" and take them to your next supervision session. Ask your manager to talk through with you what should happen in each of these situations, and what you should expect from the manager on call. The simple reply, "phone whoever is on call" is not good enough for this exercise! Get them to tell you what the person on call should do next.

Calling in specialist services

There will be times when, in order to resolve ongoing crises, you may have to call on specialist expert advice. For people with learning disabilities, this advice is most likely to be available from the Community Team for People with Learning Disabilities (CTPLD) – these used to be called Community Mental Handicap Teams (CMHT). Most CTPLDs are able to offer psychology, specialist nursing, social work, occupational therapy and speech therapy support.

• Do you know what kinds of expertise your CTPLD has available?

• Do you know how to obtain the services of the CTPLD?

Write down what you do know and how you think your service might approach the CTPLD or individuals within it. Discuss this with your line manager in supervision. Do your ideas and theirs match? Write down your discussion so that it looks like a procedure for your service to use when referring people to the CTPLD. Present it to your staff team for their ideas and comments. There you have another part of your emergency plan.

Calling in emergency services

However good your "on call" or specialist support systems may be, there will be some occasions when you need to call out the traditional emergency services: ambulance, fire brigade or even the police. Before you need to do this, find out if there is a policy or a set of guidelines in your organisation, setting out the conditions under which emergency services should be called out and who should do the calling? If there isn't, then ask your manager to give you some guidelines.

Does your organisation have good links with the local special services? Would they know what they might be expected to do if you called them out? For any situations you can think of where emergency services might be called out, write out some "briefing sheets" either for individual people or for specific situations.

You could either hand the appropriate sheet to the services as they arrive (for example, photograph and other identifying information about a person who has disappeared; important information about medication, allergies and communication skills for someone who is about to go into hospital) or staff could refer to them as required (for example to find specific ways of managing, interrupting or redirecting challenging behaviour).

Who's in charge?

Whenever you need to ask for additional help, you need to be clear about who's in charge of the situation. Whether your help is coming from a co-worker, your line management, the CTPLD or emergency services, it is probably most appropriate for you, the person who is asking for help, to stay in control and in charge directing the intervention. It is important to remember that you are asking people to help you, not asking them to take over completely.

Help can, however, take a variety of different forms, including asking people to take over for a little while so that you can have a break; asking them to instruct you in what to do; requesting that they should be organising some other resources away from the situation such as replacement furniture, extra staff. Your staying in control is particularly important when you have asked for help from outside the line management system, however difficult this might be at the time.

If you are not seen to be in charge, then your "help" will take over and start making its own decisions about what should be happening and how. It's too late to say you don't like what's happening when you've handed over responsibility. As stated earlier, you are more likely to stay in control if you

(a) ask for help before you need it, and

(b) are specific about the kind of help you want.

Here are two examples of different kinds of emergency situations, to help you think about working this way in your service. I hope that you will find these ideas on what you can do before and afterwards, useful tools for your work.

Medical emergencies

One of the commonest sources of emergencies in your service will probably have nothing to do with learning disabilities at all, but people's physical or medical needs. Accidents happen often in any home or workplace; they are just as likely to happen in services. Somebody burning themselves or cutting themselves; somebody having an epileptic fit; somebody who needs you to help them manage their diabetes, are all possible emergencies.

Before you are called upon to deal with an emergency requiring knowledge of first aid, there are a number of things you can do to check out the situation:

• What, if any, first aiding skills might you need to learn to meet people's needs (for example injecting insulin, or changing dressings?). Do you know what to do and how to do it should the situation arise?

• Is there a first aid box? Do you know where it is and what's in it? Do you know who checks it and how often? You wouldn't be the first person to go to the first aid box to get a bandage to find there was only paracetamol available.

• Do you know how to practice other first aid skills which may be required, such as putting someone into the recovery position, giving mouth to mouth resuscitation or stemming the flow of blood? If not, do you know how to get first aid training?

• Are you clear about when you would not try to deal with the situation yourself; when you would refer responsibility on either to the person's GP or by calling an ambulance?

For example, if a person is having what seem like non-stop fits, it is likely that they are in status epilepticus and you need to call an ambulance quickly. If someone has fallen over and you are not sure how to recognise if any bones have been broken, it is important that you don't move them but call an ambulance.

Be prepared

If you don't know the answers to these questions, then find out! Knowledge before or at the very beginning of a situation can avoid it developing from a relatively minor event into an emergency or a crisis. If your ignorance is shared by other staff, ask your manager to arrange

First Aid training for you.

If the service has prepared for likely emergencies by training its staff and writing specific briefing and management procedures for any specific problems for specific individuals, then you should be able to work through the emergency itself in a calm and efficient manner, directing people to help you in appropriate and pre-planned ways.

If the environment wasn't prepared, then it is likely that you will have to phone around then and there asking what to do because John has just fallen down the stairs and is lying at a funny angle. With luck, you won't do any serious damage, but luck need not have been part of the equation.

Debriefing following a medical emergency will depend on the scale of the emergency itself. Counselling someone who tried to give mouth to mouth resuscitation but without success, is different from talking through the situation where first aid was appropriately delivered and all the person needed was a few butterfly stitches on their arm.

Challenging behaviour

Working with people who you know are aggressive, or self injure, or damage their environment and so on requires a similar preparedness and debriefing procedure. Chapter 7 discusses in depth how to understand and respond to challenging behaviour. However, sometimes you have to manage new or more intense examples of people's behaviour. For this you need a well thought out range of coping strategies, so that you know what you will do even in unusual situations.

Emergencies and crises, even relating to people's behaviour, do not just appear out of nowhere. They have a beginning, a middle and an end just like any other situation. The majority of major emergencies in services result out of a series of misunderstandings by staff about what the person is trying to communicate, with or without resorting to challenging behaviour. Staff are often simply unable to understand what the person wants or doesn't want. Strategies for prevention and intervention (such as those outlined in Chapter 7) are very important.

Talking through an incident once it is over often supplies clues about how the situation developed and how to avoid it in the future. Debriefing also stops you from feeling personally to blame for what has happened, stops you developing weird and wonderful hypotheses about what was going through the person's mind (or what their intention was) at the time, and allows the whole staff team to learn for the future. It also, of course, helps identify training needs for staff and where specialist support and advice (for example from the CTPLD) may be required to guard against future emergencies.

Other emergencies - your own plans
It will be clear by now that preparation for emergency and crisis is all important. If you think through the worst possible scenarios and plan to be able to cope with them, then any situation is going to be manageable. But however many examples we work through in advance, there will always be things which take you unawares: the best you can do is minimise the number of times you are asked to cope with crises without warning or practice.

There are two skills in managing emergencies. The first is "Not letting it happen in the first place" and the second is "Learning from experience". Perhaps the Girl Guides had it right with their motto "Be Prepared"!

CHAPTER 22

Planning your career

Steve Hurry

• Take charge of your own future • Plan for the training you need to achieve what you want • Career moves and courses available

Some years ago I was working in a large establishment which closed down. I remember my thoughts on the last evening there. I had been offered three places to re-locate to and had turned down all but one. I had realised a few weeks before that I didn't have to be "spoon fed" by those in charge and just placed anywhere – I actually did have a choice. However it was not until that night that I began to look in a realistic way at some sort of career plan.

Without a plan of where I wanted to go, what I wanted to do and what I actually needed to learn, I would probably have accepted the limited options I was offered, and just drifted. Those making decisions about my future did not understand what I wanted in terms of career development, and no one else was going to care much about my career if I didn't.

Few of us, at the start of a job, look beyond the doors of the place we work, let alone plan for a future. Often we do not know what there might be beyond the doors, and anyway we are just so busy enabling and planning for people around us that we have little time to think about effective career planning for ourselves. So in this chapter I hope we can look at what sort of opportunities there are for training

and development in work involving people with learning disabilities, and how to go about planning your career.

Who decides?

We often expect management to make decisions about careers and training, and to a certain extent this is appropriate because there are implications for them in terms of the skills workers have and the likelihood of them staying. Managers do have to make decisions on priority in certain areas of staff training. This does not mean, however, that they should decide what training you get without consultation. That's your job.

Your future

So then, let's take a look at you. Here you are reading the final chapter in a book and it is on career development. I wonder if you have given any thought to your jobs over the last few years. What sort of job would you like to be doing in a year or two? Do you enjoy the work? What bits don't you like and what bits do you know are difficult? You need to ask yourself a number of questions to determine where you are and where you would like to be.

The most obvious way to progress your career is to become first a deputy and then a home leader. You can sometimes do this by gaining experience rather than formal qualifications (see Chapter 20 for details of what is involved). Often it helps to increase your skills and knowledge through courses or study, either on the care side by making sure you are up to date about services and know how to work with a range of different people with learning disabilities, or on the management side (possibly through a Certificate in Management Studies at a local college).

Planning

I know that you probably have some idea of planning services for people with learning disabilities, and setting goals. Well, the same process applies for us all in terms of career planning. Firstly, let's look at where you are now. Make a list of all the things you actually do during a day. Do you also have special responsibilities, such as being a co-worker or keyworker? Do you attend meetings on behalf of people? Have you any specific areas of knowledge or skills used in the work?

Begin to build up a picture of your strengths and include the parts of you that are not necessarily used in your work. These might be skills which are not quite related – things you learned in another job, like typing or word processing, or hobbies like cooking or photography. Having determined what your areas of strength are, make another list of areas that you know you are not so good at – and be honest! This will form the first part of your action plan towards successful career development.

Now draw up a list of both strengths and needs on a piece of paper, and leave a space for an action plan at the side. In looking at the needs you begin to find out what you need to do to go forward.

Action plan

So let's look at an Action Plan. You have acknowledged the strong areas, but what about the areas of need? Each "need area" should give you a clue about setting an action plan to develop new skills. Discuss it in supervision or with a colleague. Often you can identify training needs which can be met in the workplace or through the help of people around you. It is important to recognise that we all have skills and expertise to offer each other, whatever our position. It's not all down to managers or seniors: we all have an active part to play in training and development.

On the right is an example of the type of action plan you may wish to consider.

Make a list

Initially I want to look at making up a list of things that you can achieve. List possible training opportunities either within your workplace or at a local college. Your first list will probably consist of a lot of general ideas around things that you know you find difficult. All this is a valuable part of career planning. "Learning on the job" is the best way of learning there is but it is also important to look at more formal and theoretical training. We will look at this later on in this chapter. You can discuss, within supervision, the possibility of linking with other centres or homes to learn things that cannot be offered in your particular work setting. Don't feel constrained by the fact that your workplace doesn't seem to offer something you need to learn – you could get that help somewhere else.

Having drawn up a strengths and needs list, along with ideas for your action plan, take it to the next supervision session you have and give yourself time to discuss both your strengths and needs. Agree it with the manager or supervisor and keep a clear

STRENGTHS	NEEDS	ACTION PLAN
I am good at helping John shave.	I find that using the hoist for Bob is too difficult.	Ask Bob to show me how he'd like the hoist to be used (step by step).
I enjoy planning the menu each week.	I can't cope with the petty cash system - I always get it wrong.	Ask Julie from the office to come and give me some help.
I went on an assertiveness training course last year.	I want to develop my skills working with Bob and John, in helping them to talk about feelings.	Look at counselling course at local college.

Action plan: Look at your strengths and your training needs, then consider how the needs can be met.

record of things you need to learn or try out. This whole piece of work can be acknowledged in any appraisals that you may have, but can also be used in forming your CV (curriculum vitae) or application forms when applying for a new job.

Another important feature of meeting with your supervisor in the way described is that you both have an opportunity to set a time scale for training. It is important to do this because otherwise, what with the everyday rush in work, things will either get forgotten, or more importantly it will be forgotten that they are important!

Having looked at training needs which can be covered "on the job" - there will be some areas which cannot. Make a list of these separately and discuss with your supervisor. They may be as clear as the need to learn the recovery position and some first aid, or more complicated, like needing to understand more about difficult behaviour. Whatever it is, work out how and when this might be achieved and negotiate with your manager about releasing you. So many of us go on training days or workshops purely because it happens to be our "turn" to go or because some staff training time has to be used up. Turn the tables: start to say in advance what you want and why you want specific areas of training.

Use the people around you! People who work with you may have specific skills or knowledge or even a way of working that is helpful to you in learning more. People with learning disabilities can also show you things: they each have different skills and experiences to share with you. We often fall into the trap of being providers and "carers" for people. Sometimes we need to turn that round and look at ways in which people who use the service can help us develop more effective ways of working. This may help in developing your awareness of the views of people with learning disabilities about the services they receive, as well as your own personal development.

Formal training

What about more formal training? Perhaps your list suggests some type of studying which cannot be provided by your organisation or local authority. Most local colleges have opportunities within the adult education programme with both daytime and evening courses available. Leafing through my local prospectus I found 20 or so that could prove useful within the field of caring work. All adult education courses are part time and most are in the evening. To find out more about what is available contact your local college directly or watch for advertisements in local newspapers.

For more specific courses and specialised training workshops, there are a number of excellent organisations and centres of learning which work exclusively within the caring profession, for example Castle Priory College, organised through the Spastics Society. Contact your Staff Development Officer or Training Organiser – your manager will help you locate them. If you work in a private or voluntary organisation you may still be able to join staff in social services or the health service – it is always worth asking!

It may well be that the formal training you require is in the form of examination or assessment courses, such as GCSE, AEB or a course approved by the Central Council for Education and Training in Social Work (CCETSW). In this case the local college isn't always the best route. For GCSE or AEB it may be, but there are opportunities at other learning centres and also through correspondence courses.

Whichever you choose, seek the help of those who organise and run the courses themselves: they're always ready to help you find the most appropriate training.

Social work

Formal training in social work is changing. By 1995 the CQSW (Certificate of Qualification in Social Work) will be replaced with a new qualification called the DipSW (Diploma in Social Work). In terms of professional training this is the qualification you will need to work at different levels within the statutory authorities (social services), and in many voluntary and charitable organisations too. It will be the only method of entry to work as a qualified social worker Any course should be approved by CCETSW, so when you apply remember to check that it is an approved course.

To get on to a CQSW/DipSW course you will need to have gained academic success in GCSE A levels, and you may have a degree. If you are over 25 or so it may be acceptable to apply without any academic qualifications, but you will need to have some form of social work experience like the work you are now doing, or some type of voluntary work. About half of all entrants to the existing CQSW courses are "mature" students and half from colleges or university.

The course usually lasts two years and combines work placement with theoretical training. In some cases it can be a three year part time course, which may suit those with family commitments. The Open University (OU) and some polytechnics plan to organise the course through a mixture of full time and part time learning. Information from the OU.

Mental handicap nursing

The other main route for "qualifying" training in learning disability services is the Registered Nurse in Mental Handicap (RNMH) qualification. This enables you to work as a specialist nurse within the NHS (hospitals), staffed housing or similar (nursing homes, day services, specialist units, etc). If you do not have the five GCSEs required for entrance you can sit a special entrance test.

Training placements are with people with learning disabilities within hospital and community settings, However, the nursing qualification, especially on new Project 2000 courses, entitles you to work with all age groups and is acceptable outside the NHS as an equivalent professional qualification.

For information on other related professions in the field of learning disability, national contact addresses are listed in the Resources section that follows this chapter.

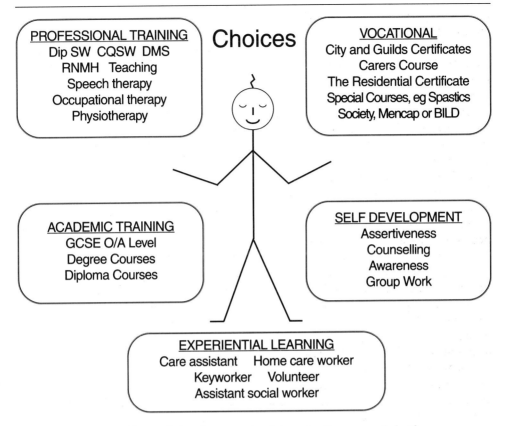

Which of the many different choices for career development suits your needs best?

Most colleges have courses designed for the caring professions, and there is a whole range of City and Guilds certificate courses from basic care practice to advanced management training. Other similar courses include some on "care in the community" and the Residential Care Certificate organised through local colleges. There are also courses organised through large agencies such as Mencap, the Spastics Society and the British Institute of Learning Disabilities (BILD), which are often based in local colleges.

The best way to find out what is available is to spend some time at the local reference library, or approach colleges and polytechnics. Most produce a prospectus of courses annually, and fees are always reasonable.

Branching out

Taking a look at the local paper last week I saw there were a number of interesting and different vocational, educational and leisure type courses being run at my local college. I studied last year on a counselling course at the local college and I learned a great deal about how the theory could help with my practice. It did not lead to a formal qualification but I now use it in my work with people with learning disabilities and can add it to any future application form or CV.

More importantly, going back to the strengths and needs lists I produced last year for myself, it turned what in fact was a "weakness" into a "strength". You may need to think, as I did, about having a mixture of vocational courses (such as assertiveness training, counselling, group work, etc) and more formal or theoretical training (GCSE, Diploma or Degree courses). Many people find they cannot get time off to study at college or polytechnic. If so, you may wish to consider a correspondence course.

The Open University

The main distinguishing feature of the Open University is that each course has a fixed starting date, gives tutorial support, has a mixture of assessment/examination and works flexibly with a lot of different ways of enabling learning. The OU holds residential courses and workshops and gives a certificate on the successful completion of each course.

There are a variety of different relevant courses you can take with the OU. They have an extensive list of courses designed for the caring professions, available from the University's Department of Health and Social Welfare. The real benefit of this way of learning is that you can spread it over a number of years and eventually, through each certificate you get, build up credits towards a full degree or diploma. A fair amount of the courses are work related and some expect you to undertake a project around your existing job. The OU may also be able to help you with funding through grants and bursaries.

Vocational qualifications

The National Vocational Qualification (NVQ) system offers a new approach to all types of vocational qualifications currently being introduced, and they are likely to become standard requirements for all employment in the future.

NVQs represent a radical departure from existing qualifications, as they are based on nationally agreed, employment led standards of competence, and are primarily assessed in the workplace or involve workplace activities.

The NVQ system is not yet fully in place. In the case of the caring professions the work is still being piloted and monitored and may still be a number of years away. However, it is worth indicating just how this will affect you in the future:

The qualifications making up NVQ will be set at graded levels of skill and competency. They are designed so that people who wish to transfer jobs can take their past skills/training and experience with them in a way that is clear and acceptable to every employer.

There are within the NVQ both practical and theoretical tasks to complete, and until you have proved your competence in the areas laid down you will not be able to pass on to higher grades of NVQ. There is a mixture of self assessment, manager assessment and external assessment involved in NVQ and it is designed to be as fair and comprehensive as possible.

Your action plan

1. Get some idea of where you are and where you want to be.
2. Make a list of what you feel are your strengths, and your needs.
3. Set some goals: what do you need to learn or experience?
4. Start an action plan going – time scales are important.
5. Involve others and get their ideas and help too.

Useful contacts
See also Resources section on pages 173-174.

CCETSW, Derbyshire House, St Chad Street, London WC1H 8AD. Tel: 071 278 2455.
City and Guilds, 46 Brittania Street, London WC1X 9RG. Tel: 071 278 2468.
Open University, Information Office, Department of Health and Social Welfare, Milton Keynes, MK7 6AA. Tel: 0908 653743.

Resources

Voluntary organisations

ASBAH (Association for Spina Bifida and Hydrocephalus), Asbah House, 42 Park Road, Peterborough PE1 2UQ. Tel: 01733 555988.

Association of Swimming Therapy, 26 Stone Grove, Edgware HA8 7UA. Tel: 0181 958 1642.

British Epilepsy Association, Anstey House, 40 Hanover Square, Leeds LS3 1BE. Tel: 0113 2439393. **National Information Centre – Helpline 0345 089599** (local call charge only).

British Sports Association for the Disabled, Mary Glen Haig Suite, Solecast House, 13-27 Brunswick Place, London N1 6DX. Tel: 0171 490 4919.

Carers National Association, 20-25 Glasshouse Yard, London EC1A 4JS. 0171 490 8818.

Commission for Racial Equality, Elliot House, 10-12 Allington St, London SW1E 5EH. Tel: 0171 828 7022.

Disabled Living Foundation, 380-384 Harrow Rd, London W9 2HU. Tel: 0171 289 6111.

Down's Syndrome Association, 155 Mitcham Rd, London SW17 9PG. Tel: 0181 682 4001.

Incontinence Advisory Service, Disability North at the Dene Centre, Castle Farm Road, Newcastle-upon-Tyne NE3 1PH. Helpline: 0191 213 0050.

International Cerebral Palsy Society, c/o 19 St Mary's Grove, Chiswick, London W4 3LL. Tel: 0181 995 5721.

MENCAP, Royal Society for Mentally Handicapped Children and Adults, 123 Golden Lane, London EC1Y 0RT. Tel: 0171 454 0454.

National Association for the Protection from Sexual Abuse of Adults and Children with Learning Disabilities (NAPSAC), Pam Cooke, Dept Learning Disabilities, University of Nottingham Medical School, Queen's Medical Centre, Nottingham NG7 2UH.

National Autistic Society, 276 Willesden Lane, London NW2 5RB. Tel: 0181 451 1114.

National Citizen Advocacy, Unit 2K, Leroy House, 436 Essex Road, N1 3QP.

National Deaf-Blind and Rubella Association, (SENSE), 11-13 Clifton Terrace, Finsbury Park London N4 3SR. Tel: 0171 272 7774.

National Society for Epilepsy, Chalfont St Peter, Gerrards Cross, Buckinghamshire SL9 0RJ. Tel: 01494 873991.

Riding for the Disabled Association, Avenue 'R', National Agricultural Centre, Kenilworth, Warwickshire CV8 2LY. Tel: 01203 696510.

Royal National Institute for the Blind, 224 Great Portland St, London W1N 6AA. Tel: 0171 388 1266.

Royal National Institute for the Deaf, 105 Gower St, London WC1E 6AH. Tel: 0171 387 8033.

Values into Action (Learning Disabilities), Oxford House, Derbyshire St, London E2 6HG.

Professional bodies

British Association for Counselling, 1 Regent Place, Rugby, Warwicks CV21 2PJ. Tel: 01788 578328/9.

British Association of Art Therapists, 11a Richmond Road, Brighton BN2 3RL.

British Association of Occupational Therapists, 6-8 Marshalsea Rd, Southwark, London SE1 1HL. Tel: 0171 357 6480.

British Psychological Society, St Andrew's House, 48 Princess Rd East, Leicester LE1 7DR. Tel: 0116 2549568.

British Society for Music Therapy, 69 Avondale Avenue, East Barnet, Herts EN4 8NB. Tel: 0181 368 8879.

Central Council for Education and Training in Social Work (CCETSW), Derbyshire House, St Chad Street, London WC1H 8AD. Tel: 0171 278 2455.

Chartered Society of Physiotherapy, 14 Bedford Row, London WC1R 4ED. Tel: 0171 242 1941.

College of Speech and Language Therapists, 7 Bath Place, Rivington Street, London EC2A 3DR. Tel: 0171 613 3855.

Disablement Employment Advisers – contact the Department of Employment.

National Council for Special Education, York House, Exhall Grange, Wheelwright Lane,

Coventry CV7 9HP. Tel: 01203 362414.
Royal College of Nursing of the UK, 20 Cavendish Square, London W1M 0AB. Tel: 071 409 3333.
Social Care Association, 23a Victoria Rd, Surbiton, Surrey KT6 4JZ. Tel: 081 390 6831/4639.

Education and training

British Institute of Learning Disabilities, Wolverhampton Road, Kidderminster, Worcestershire DY10 3PP. Tel: 01562 850251.
City and Guilds, 46 Brittania Street, London WC1X 9RG. Tel: 0171 278 2468.
King's Fund Centre, 126 Albert St, London NW1 7NF. Tel: 0171 267 6112.
Open University, Information Office, Department of Health and Social Welfare, Milton Keynes, MK7 6AA. Tel: 01908 653743.
National Council for Vocational Qualifications (NCVQ), 222 Euston Road, London NW1 2BZ. Tel: 0171 387 9898.
Pavilion Publishing (Brighton) Ltd, 8 St George's Place, Brighton, East Sussex BN1 4GB. Tel: 01273 623222. *Training materials.*
SCOPE, 12 Park Crescent, London W1. Tel: 0171 636 5020.
Tizard Centre, Dr Hilary Brown, Beverley Farm, University of Kent, Canterbury, Kent CT2 7LZ. Tel: 0227 764000

Publications

Professor Karen Luker, **Health and Social Care in the Community,** Whelan Building, University of Liverpool, PO Box 147, Liverpool L69 3BX.
Professor Len Barton, **Disability & Society,** Division of Education, University of Sheffield, Sheffield S10 2TN.
Professor W I Fraser, Editor, **Journal of Intellectual Disability Research,** 55 Park Place, Cardiff CF1 3AT.
Care Weekly Magazine, 9 White Lion St, London N1 9XJ. Tel: 071 837 8727.
Community Care Magazine, Quadrant Hse, Sutton, Surrey SM2 5AS. Tel: 081 652 4861.
Disability Rights Handbook, The Disability Alliance Educational and Research Association,

Universal House, 88-94 Wentworth St, London E1 7SA. Tel: 071 247 8776.
British Journal of Learning Disability (MH)/Mental Handicap Research (MHR), BILD Publications, Bank House, 8A Hill Road, Clevedon, Bristol BS21 7HH. Tel: 0272 343096.

Research and evaluation

Department of Social Policy, Leeds University LS2 9JT.
Tizard Centre, Beverley Farm, University of Kent, Canterbury, Kent CT2 7LZ. Tel: 0227 764000
Hester Adrian Research Centre, University of Manchester, Manchester M13 9PL.
Norah Fry Research Centre, 3 Priory Road, Bristol BS8 1TX.
Department of Learning Disabilities, The University of Nottingham, Floor E, South Block, University Hospital, Nottingham NG7 2UH.
National Development Team, St Peter's Court, 8 Trumpet Street, Manchester M1 5LW.
Professor David Felce, **Mental Handicap in Wales,** Applied Research Unit, 55 Park Place, Cardiff CF1 3AT.
Professor James Hogg, White Top Centre, Social Work Department, **University of Dundee,** Dundee DD1 4HN.
Professor Sheila Hollins, **St George's Hospital Medical School,** Department of Mental Health Sciences, Jenner Wing, Cranmer Terrace, London SW17 0RE.
Professor Chris Cullen, **University of St Andrews,** Psychological Laboratory, St Andrews, Fife, Scotland KY16 9JU.

Advocacy

Dr Richard Wood, **British Council for Organisations of Disabled People (BCODP),** Victoria Buildings, 117 High Street, Clay Cross, Derbyshire.
People First, Instrument House, 207-215 Kings Cross Rd, London WC1X 9DB. Tel: 071 713 6400.
National Citizen Advocacy, Unit 2K, Leroy House, 436 Essex Road, N1 3QP.

Index